Colour Therapy for Love & Romance

by
Rochie Rana
(India's First Certified Colour Therapist)

Editor
Mrs. Gita Nath

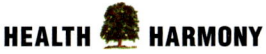

An imprint of
B. Jain Publishers (P) Ltd.
USA - EUROPE - INDIA
www.bjainbooks.com

COLOUR THERAPY FOR LOVE AND ROMANCE

First Edition: 2009

All rights reserved. No part of this book may be reproduced, stored in a retrieval system or transmitted, in any form or by any means, mechanical, photocopying, recording or otherwise, without any prior written permission of the publisher.

© with the author

Published by Kuldeep Jain for

HEALTH HARMONY

An imprint of
B. JAIN PUBLISHERS (P) LTD.
An ISO 9001 : 2000 Certified Company
1921/10, Chuna Mandi, Paharganj, New Delhi 110 055 (INDIA)
Tel.: 91-11-2358 0800, 2358 1100, 2358 1300, 2358 3100
Fax: 91-11-2358 0471 • *Email:* info@bjain.com
Website: **www.bjainbooks.com**

Cover design & layout: Vijesh Chahal

Printed in India by
J.J. OFFSET PRINTERS
522, FIE, Patpar Ganj, Delhi - 110 092
Tel.: 91-11-2216 9633, 2215 6128

ISBN: 978-81-319-0541-8

Publisher's note

From the name immemorial colour therapy is being used by man-kind as a powerful therapy. It is a truly holistic, non-invasive & healing therapy which dates back to thousands of years. Colour is a simple light of varying wavelengths and frequencies. Colours affect our lives in many ways, from our choice of eating, to clothes, to our habits.

It affects our mood as blue is calming-red is aggressive. We use colours depending on our moods as well, but are unaware of it. Here is a digest by Rochie Rana, India's first colour therapist on usage of colours for love & romance. There is so much of romance & love that can be added to our lives simply by using different colours. Use these tips & see the difference for yourself.

– Kuldeep Jain
CEO

Dedication

This book is dedicated to my parents, for encouraging me at every stage of my life, from studying curious subjects such as colour therapy to allowing me to be the wanderer, that I have reached so far…

And ofcourse, to my brothers for all the love they have given me and for being the greatest strength of my life!

Acknowledgement

This book would have remained a daunting task if it wasn't for my friend Gautam Chintamani who encouraged me to pursue colour therapy relentlessly. Also, Mr. Anil Srivatsa and Meow FM for being a ceaseless learning colour ground and the entire team of Radio Today for their continual support.

And then walking down the lanes of my memory, for Ginnie and Rajjat, two friends without whose constant attention and love, this book would have taken twice as long to be completed and ofcourse for the love that I have found and lost many times in the heart of the Himalayas.

Preface

If there is an emotion in this world that encompasses fire and cold, tenderness and shadows, it is love.

This one emotion has inspired poets and artists across centuries to craft their masterpieces and to immortalize their loves.

Colour therapy for love and romance is an endeavour to try and add more colour to love than it already possesses.

Love brings with it, many emotions; it makes you crave, its warmth steals the calmness that lies within your heart. Love gives and in turn asks for more, making it a relentless circle of loving and loathing and it is then that we often find ourselves looking for answers. This book tries to make every phase of love and gives more wonderful and magnificent approach with the help of colours and its appropriate use.

Here is something that reflects the emotions to which every lover goes through:

>Gathering oblivion and butterflies
>The Venus night glowed outside
>The windowpane;
>While youth and memories
>Rested in my hair.
>The air is thick with the familiarity
>Of knowing you were never apart
>Yet I tumble over pebbles
>And separation tonight
>My fortitude goes planting flags
>In the hidden corners of love for you

I love you like a clumsy girl in spring
You are everywhere
In the golden wheat
In the blazing war
In the delicate sound of a guitar
In the thick weeks that make a lifetime
While my mad heart
Gathers oblivion and butterflies
With the Venus night tonight.

All the best to those who have the courage to fall in love and take what it brings with it and wishes of valor upon those who are still walking in the shadows, afraid to embrace the sunlight that love is!

— Rochie Rana

Author's note

It is hoped that this book will prove to be a source of inspiration for many, for finding true love, having the conviction to make relationships work, dealing with the painful moments of heartbreak and for finding the strength to look beyond past hurt, possessing the courage to move forth in life with the knowledge that love awaits at every corner in the journey of life and the day we are ready to embrace love, love will be waiting for you with arms wide open.

I hold it true from In Memoriam

'I hold it true, whate'er befall;

I feel it, when I sorrow most;

'T' is better to have loved and lost

Than never to have loved at all'

Lord Alfred Tennyson- 1809-92

- Rochie Rana

Contents

1. **INTRODUCING COLOURS** — 1
   - Understanding colour — 5
   - History — 7
   - The colour spectrum — 9
   - Colour Terminology — 11
     - Hue
     - Tint
     - Shade
     - Value
     - Intensity
   - Colour Scheme — 13
     - Monochromatic
     - Monochromentary
     - Triadic
   - Colour: Characteristics and effects — 15
     - Red
     - Orange
     - Yellow
     - Green
     - Blue
     - Indigo
     - violet
   - Using this book — 21

2. **INTERIORS FOR SINGLES** — 24
   - Colours you wear — 29
   - Food for love — 34
   - Flowers and candles — 35
   - Suitable fragrances — 37
   - Colours in nature — 39

3. **THE FIRST DATE** — 40
   - The first date — 44
     - Attire colours for women
     - The perfect lip colour
     - Ideal fragrances
     - Attire colours for men
     - Flowers for the first date
     - The first date and dinner

4. **KNOW YOUR PARTNER THROUGH HIS FAVOURITE COLOURS** — 52
     - White
     - Purple
     - Blue
     - Green
     - Yellow
     - Orange
     - Red
     - Pink
     - Brown
     - Grey
     - Black

5. **COLOUR COMPATIBILITY** — 65
     - Red and white
     - Red and violet
     - Red and blue

- Red and green
- Red and orange
- Red and pink
- Red and brown
- Red and black
- White and purple
- White and blue
- White and green
- White and yellow
- White and orange
- White and pink
- White and brown
- White and black
- Purple and blue
- Purple and green
- Purple and yellow
- Purple and orange
- Purple and pink
- Purple and brown
- Purple and black
- Blue and green
- Blue and orange
- Blue and pink
- Brown and blue
- Blue and black
- Green and yellow
- Green and orange
- Green and pink
- Green and brown
- Green and black
- Yellow and orange
- Yellow and pink
- Yellow and brown
- Yellow and Black
- Orange and pink
- Orange and brown
- Orange and black
- Pink and brown
- Pink and black
- Brown and black

6. **TOWARDS A HEALTHY AND BEAUTIFUL RELATIONSHIP** — 103
   Step 1: Discover the joys of communication — 104
   - Communication — 105
   Step 2: The ultimate commitment: Sharing your inner self — 116
   - Chilli hot chocolate — 121
   Step 3: Merging spiritually — 122
   - Golden fried eggplant spread — 128
   Step 4: More than sex — 133

7. **BREAKING UP** — 145

Chapter 1
INTRODUCING COLOURS

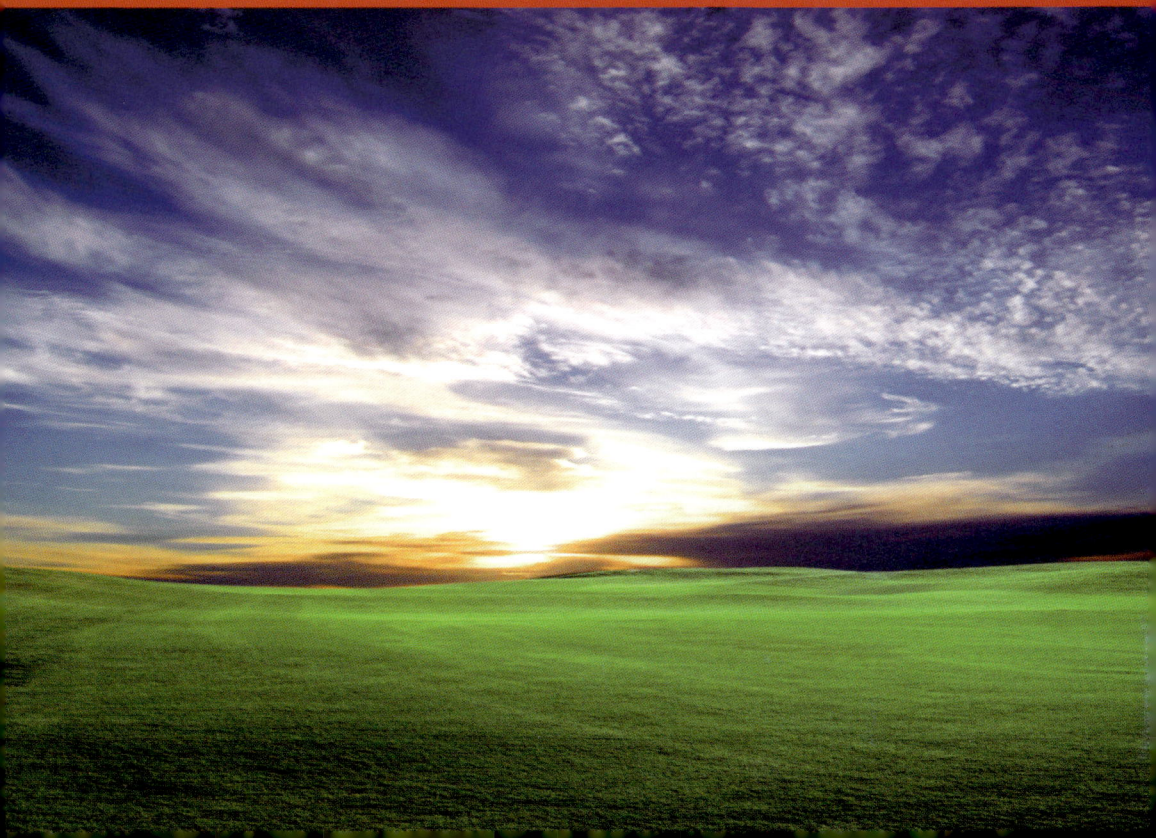

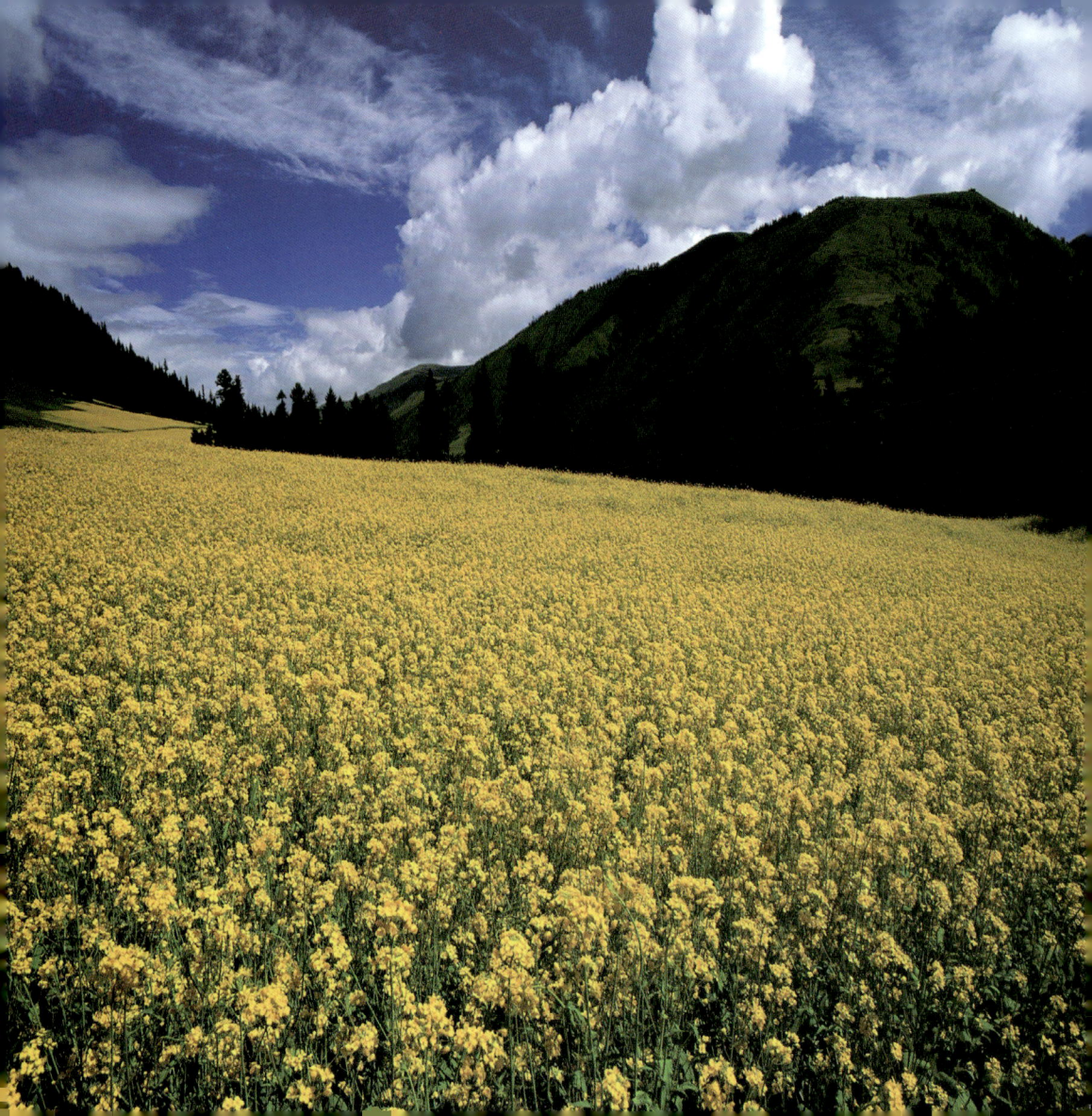

Introducing Colours

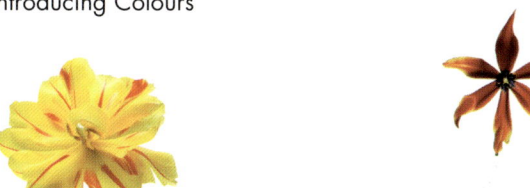
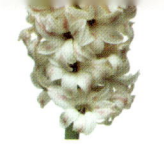
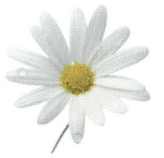

'Nature's first green is gold, Her hardest hue to hold.
Her early leaf's a flower, But only so for an hour.
Then leaf subsides to leaf, So Eden sank to grief.
So dawn goes down to day, Nothing gold can stay.'

– *Robert Frost*

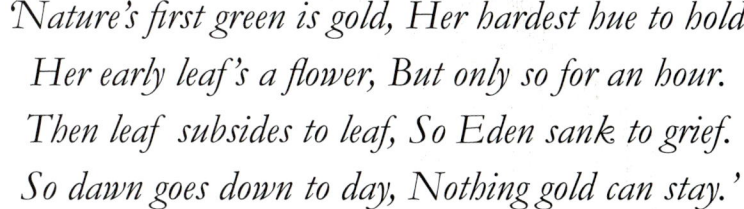
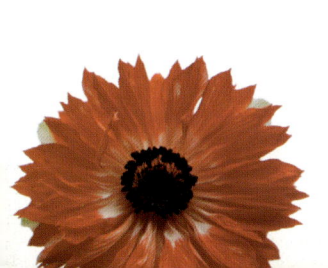
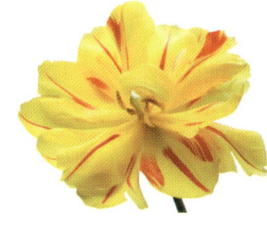
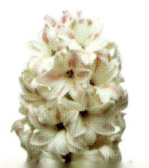

Poets and artists have, since time immemorial, best expressed themselves through the metaphor of colour. Colours are not merely the tools of an artist but are all pervasive. They enrich our experiences of life and give it a meaning. Isaac Mizarani very rightly says, 'Colour is like food for the spirit-plus it's not addictive or fattening.'

Colour first touches human life at the very time of conception. At birth, man is greeted by all shades of colours and thereafter, it becomes a constant in his life.

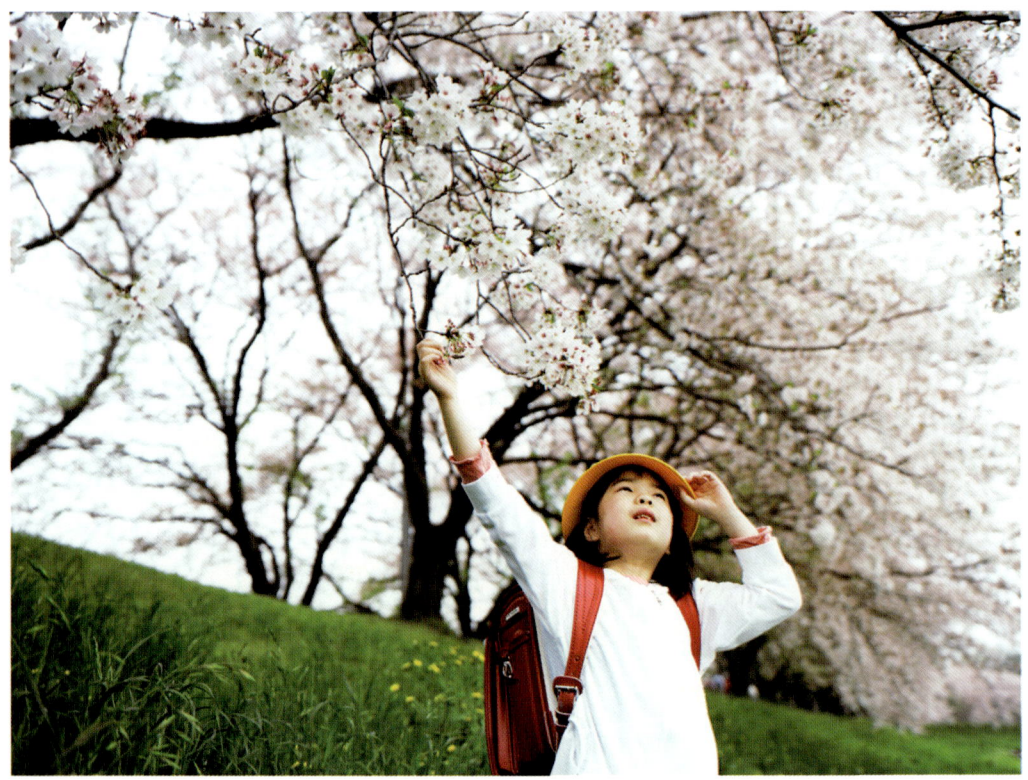

Understanding Colour

Colour comprises rays of light which has a huge spectrum ranging from microwaves to cosmic rays. Only a narrow band of energy, placed roughly in the middle of the electromagnetic spectrum of light, is visible to the human eye.

Light is made up of rays some of which aren't visible to the naked eye. All rays have different energies, frequencies and wavelengths which determine colour.

Colour depends on what parts of the rays are absorbed by the object on which they fall. Therefore, a rose appears red as, all other energies, except red, which are weaker, get absorbed by the flower. Only the colour 'red' bounces back, giving the rose a red colour.

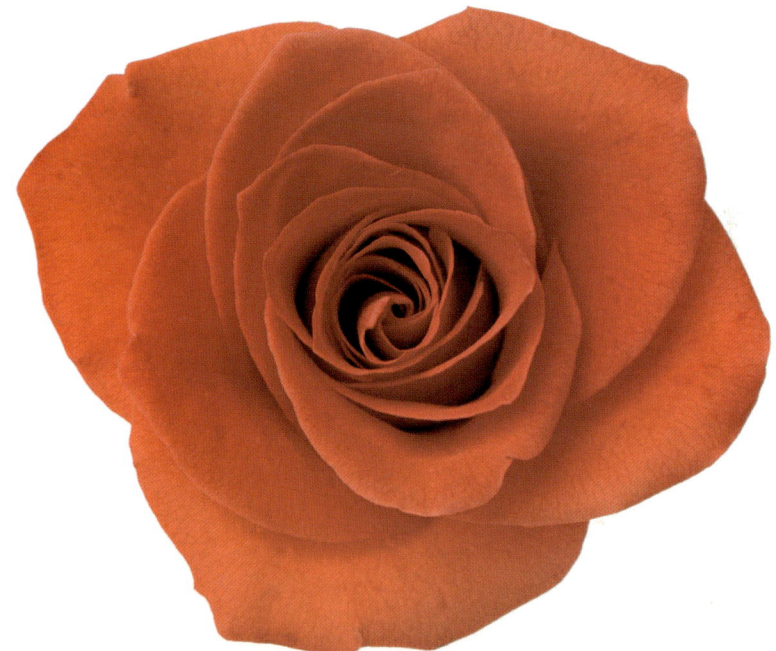

Colour Therapy for Love & Romance

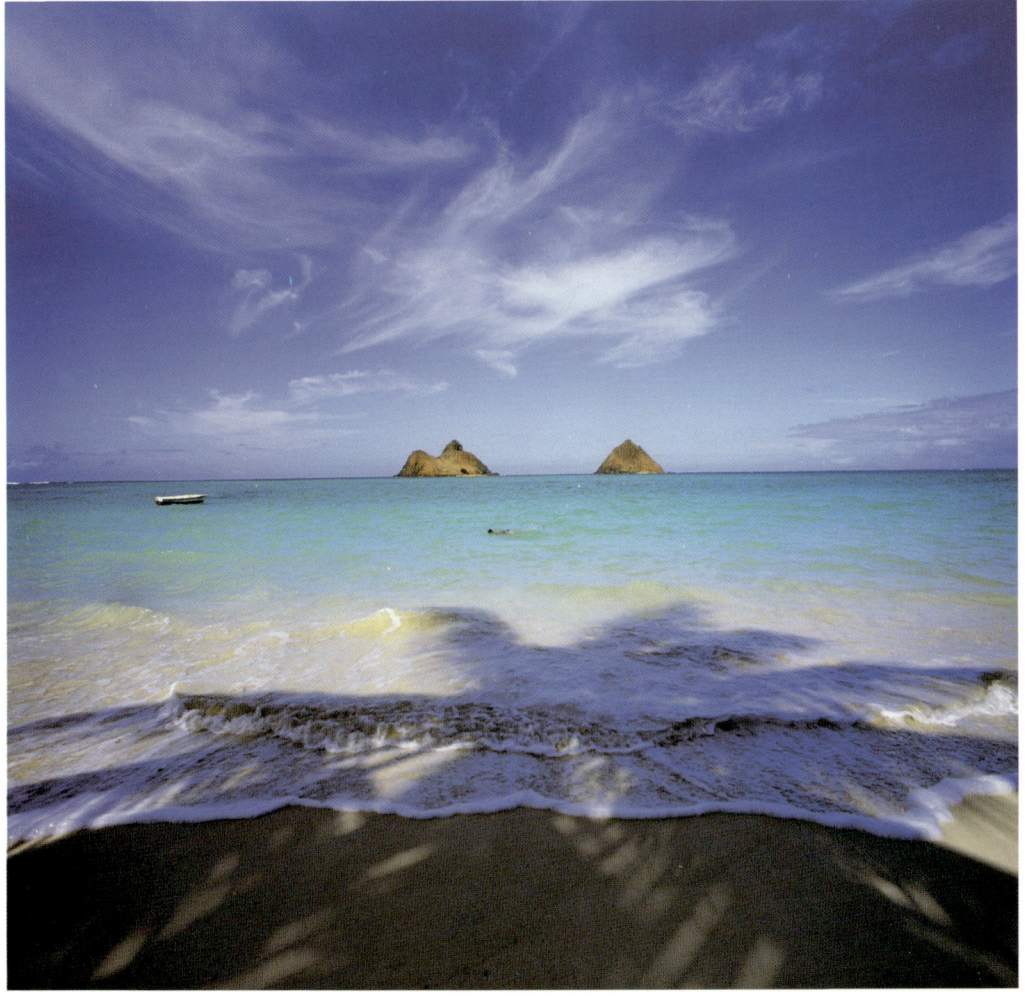

The energy of the rays, which determines colour, also transfers a certain amount of energy to the one who perceives the colour and subtly influences the state of the person's mind and body. It is a well known and accepted fact that merely looking at colours like orange, yellow and red puts one's body in the active and energetic mode; while colours like blue and green relax and soothe the mind.

This visible spectrum of light has been used to heal people physically and mentally since ancient times. This form of alternative healing is known as Chromotherapy or colour therapy.

History

Chromotherapy is not a recent invention but can be traced back to centuries. India, China and Greece had been practising it effectively even when they weren't aware of the scientific principles behind the healing processes.

The Egyptians, in accordance with their hermetic traditions, built temples which were adorned with colours. They were used as sanctuaries for the ailing where the sick were immersed in coloured light for a specific period of time. The Greeks used colour-specific minerals, stones and crystals to heal different ailments.

The ancient Chinese medical practitioners effectively used colours to cure people. The Chinese medical text, 'Nei Ching', dating back nearly 2000 years, states how one's health can be ascertained by reading the colour and appearance of the skin, tissues and organs.

Ayurveda and Chromotherapy have coexisted in India. Ayurvedacharyas believed that the human body has seven energy centres, 'Chakras'. Each 'Chakra' corresponds to a particular colour of the spectrum. The ailing were treated by establishing a balance and harmony in the energies of the body, using seven colours.

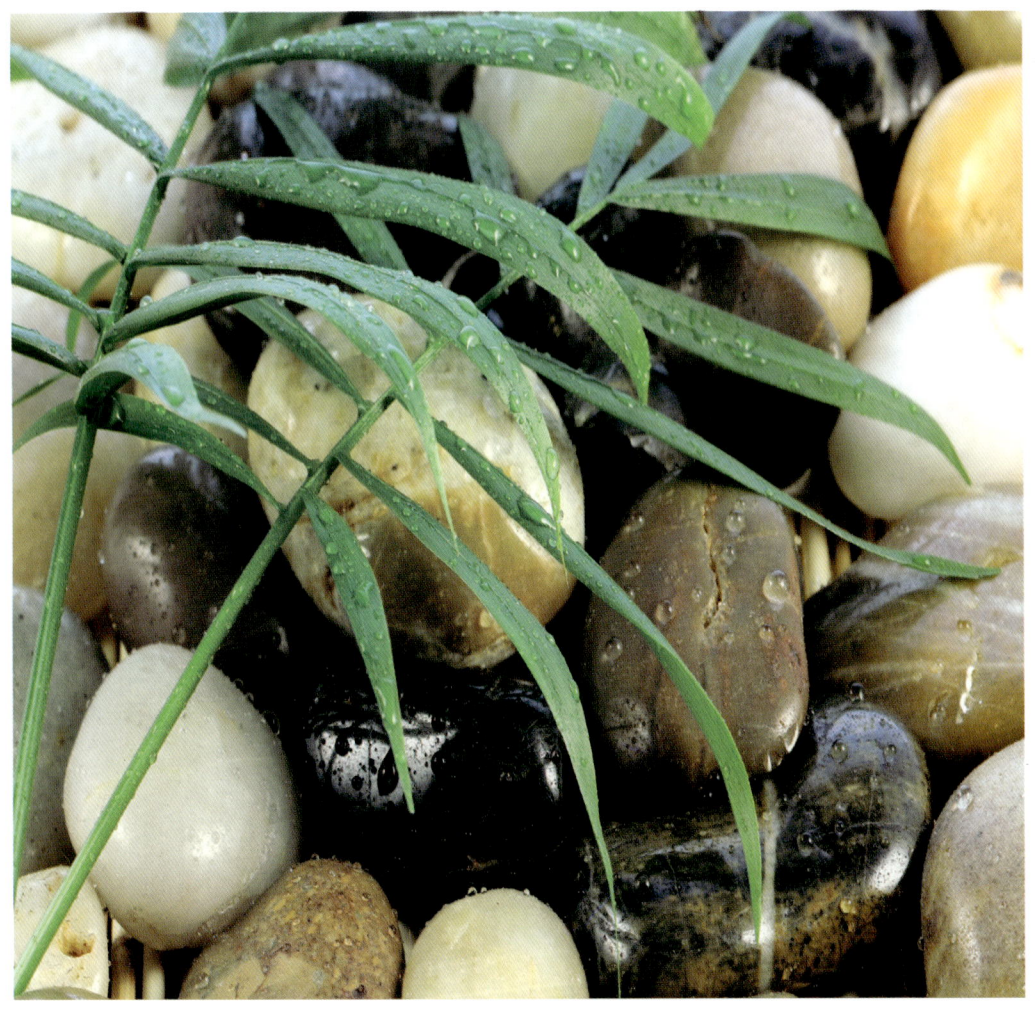

Introducing Colours

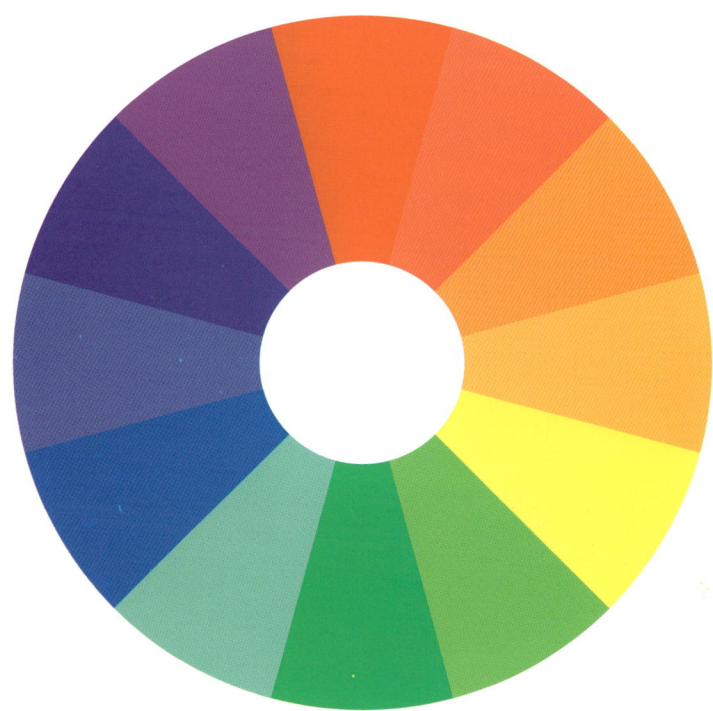

The Colour Spectrum

The spectrum of light consists of three primary colours– Red, Yellow and Blue. These cannot be created by mixing other colours.

The Secondary colours namely Orange, Green and Violet are obtained by mixing equal parts of two primary colours.

Tertiary colours are produced by combining equal parts of primary and secondary colours. When these are further mixed with White or Black, quaternary colours are obtained.

Isaac Newton observed this spectrum of light and colours and formulated the Colour Wheel.

In this, he placed the three primary colours equidistant around the perimeter of the circle. Then he evenly placed the secondary colours obtained by mixing the primary colours, adjacent to the primary colours.

Newton went further and associated each colour of the wheel with a specific musical note. A century after Newton's formulation of the colour wheel, Johann Wolfgang von Goethe attached psychological effects to the colours. He created a wheel which was divided into two- the positive and the negative. The positive part consisted of colours from Red, through Orange to Yellow which are cheerful in nature. The negative part had colours that ran from Green through Violet to Blue regarded as weak and disconcerting colours.

Colour, as we understand it today, was developed by a Swiss colour and art theorist, Johannes Itten who modified Newton's colour wheel using Red, Yellow and Blue as the primary colours and twelve other hues. What gave his theory an edge over the previous one was the fact that he didn't consider colour merely as the physics of light but believed that each colour had inherent characteristics, which affected each individual in a psychological and spiritual way.

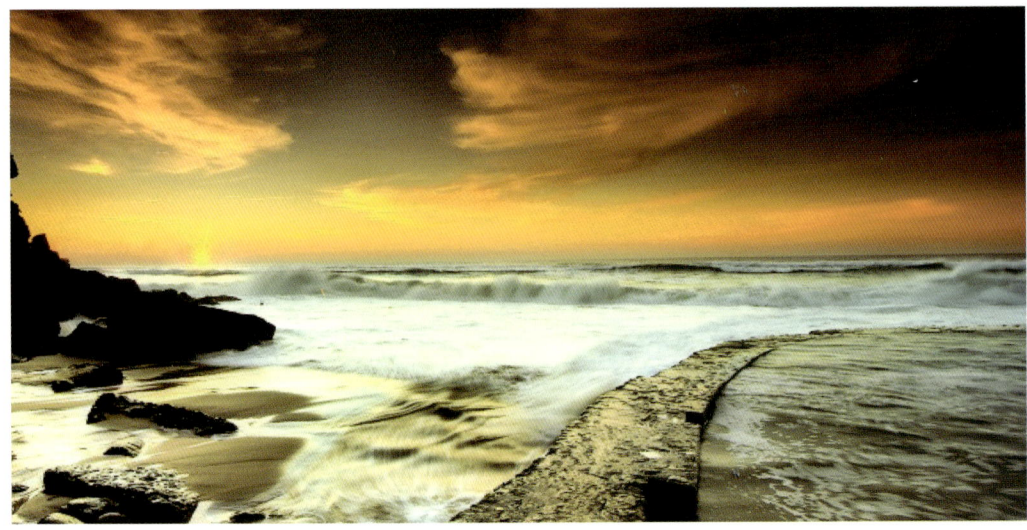

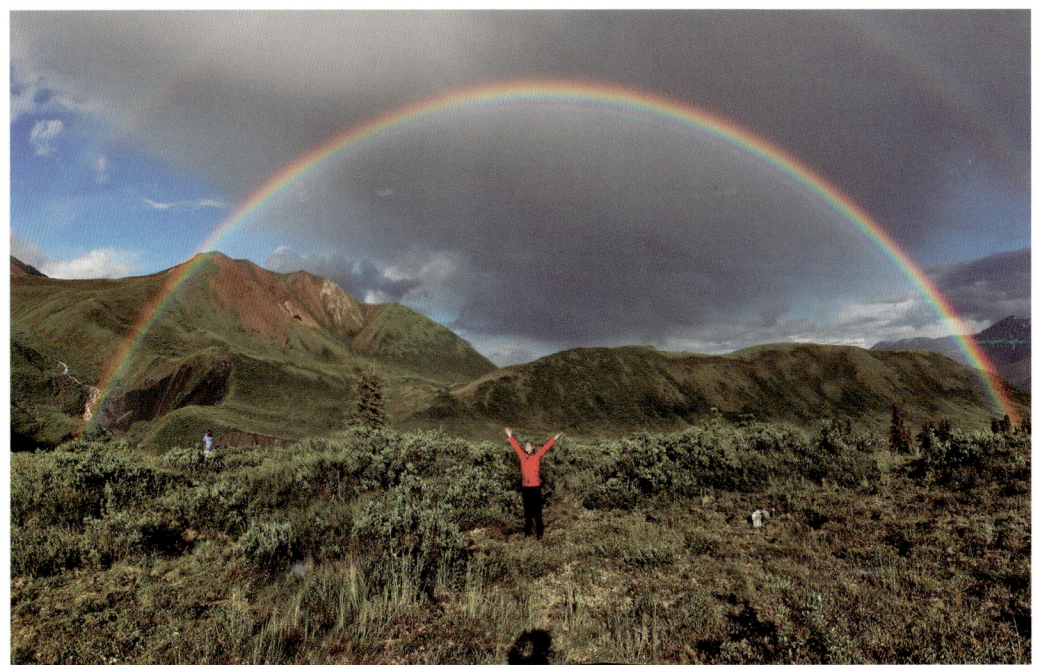

Colour Terminology

The study of colour brings with it a certain jargon that helps us in a better understanding of the various facets of colours and their combinations. Some are highly technical, meant for artists and designers while others are simple and used in common parlance.

Hue:

Hue is a synonym for colour. Every different wavelength of light produces a different colour and this is referred to as hue. There are seven hues – Violet, Indigo, Blue, Green, Yellow, Orange and Red.

Tint:

A tint is achieved by adding white to a colour. Pastel colours are obtained in this way. For example pink is a tint of red, lilac is a tint of purple.

Shade:

Just as a tint is achieved by adding white to a colour, shade is obtained with a hint of black added to a colour. For example, crimson is a shade of red and royal purple is a shade of violet.

Value:

The value of a hue indicates the relative darkness or lightness of a colour juxtaposed to other colours. For example, green has a higher value than purple.

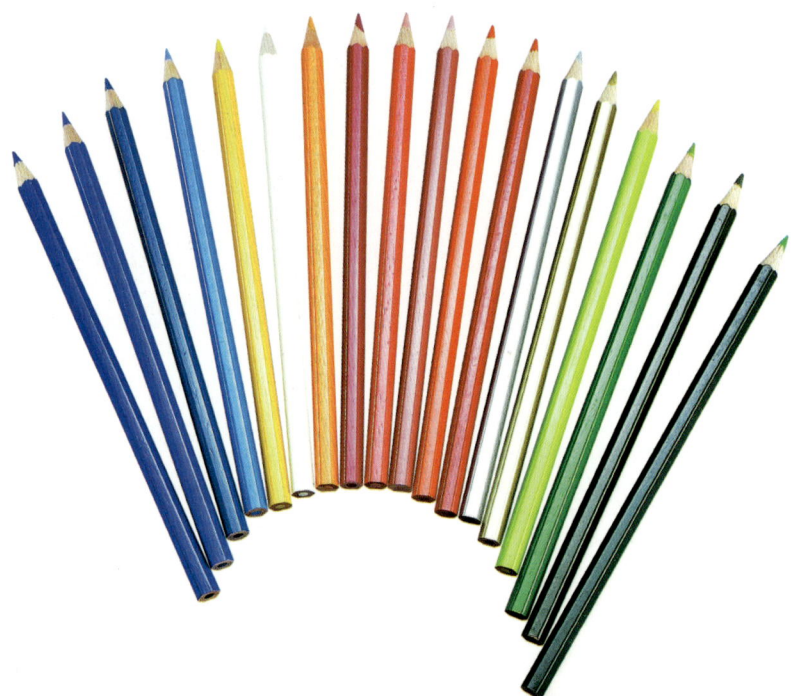

Intensity:

The intensity or saturation of a colour refers to its brightness. When a colour is not mixed with either black or white, it is considered to be at its full intensity.

Colour Scheme

Colour schemes can be incorporated in one's life to enhance its beauty and to harmonize it. These colour schemes have also been advocated by artists and designers. Some of these colour schemes are:

Monochromatic:

The use of only one colour with variation in its value, shade or tint.

Analogous:

The use of two colours, placed adjacent to each other on the colour wheel; for instance, orange and red or blue and green.

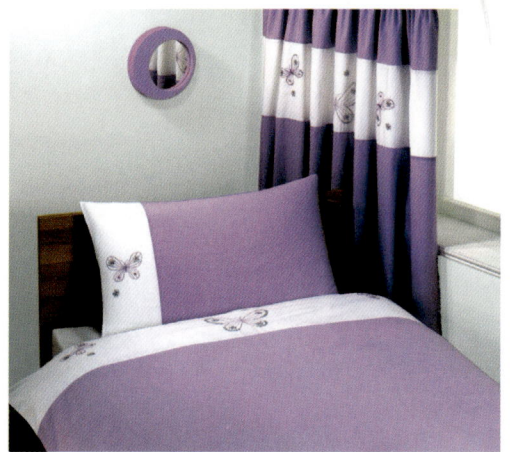

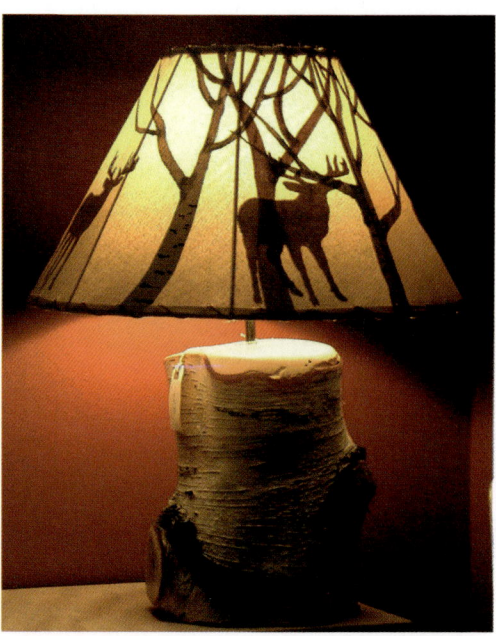

Complementary:

The use of two colours placed opposite to each other on the colour wheel; for instance, orange and blue or yellow and violet.

Triadic:

The use of three colours that are uniformly spaced on the colour wheel; for example, green, red and yellow.

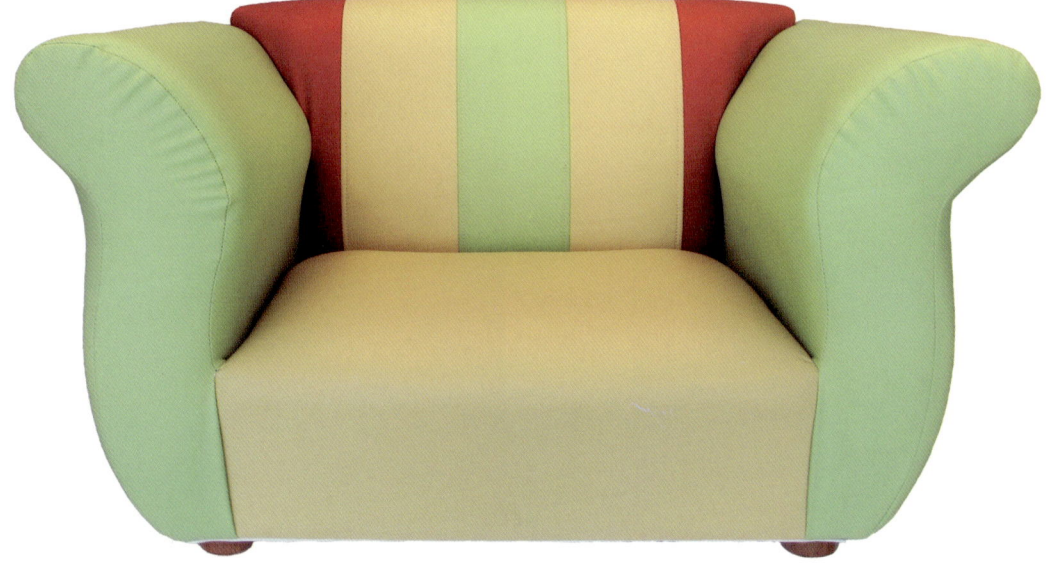

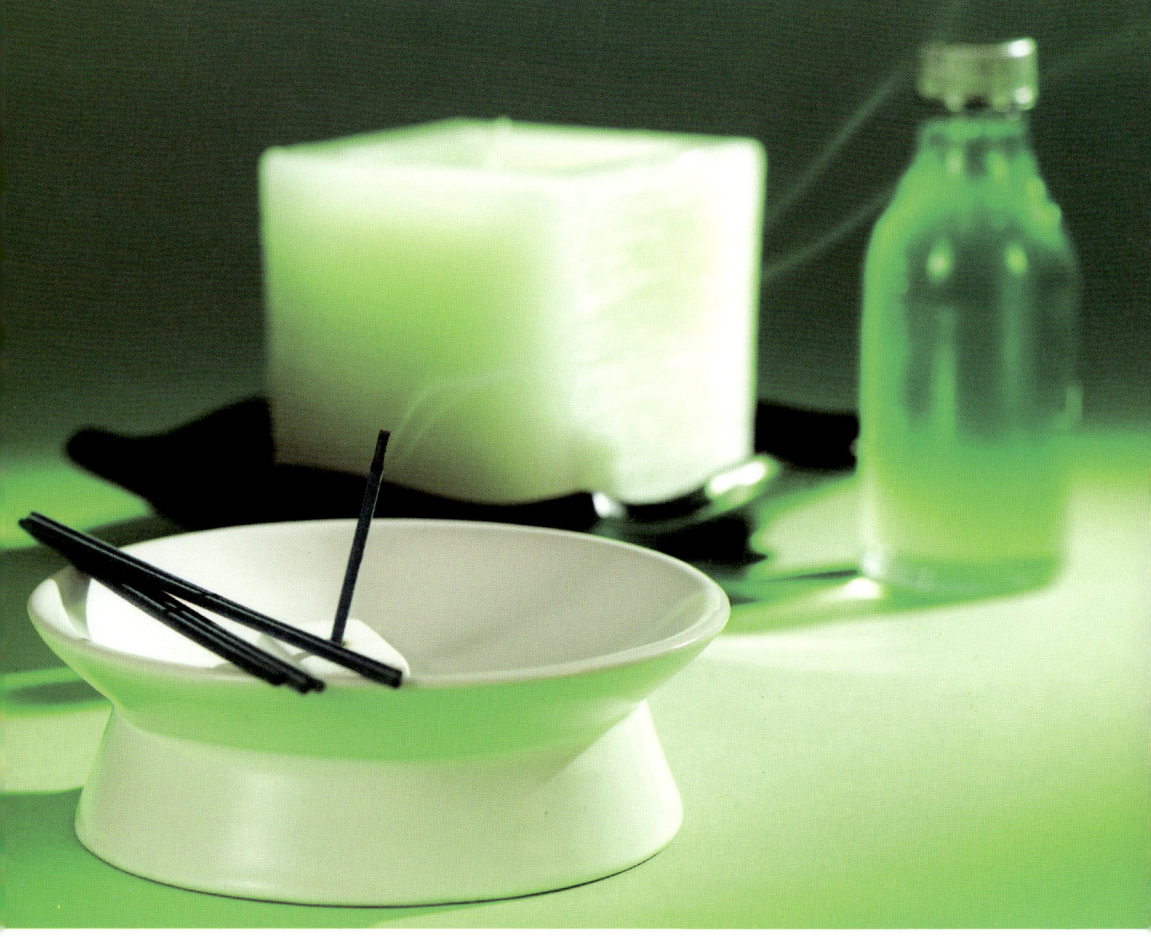

COLOUR: Characteristics and Effects

All the seven colours used in Chromotherapy have a specific physical and psychological effect on people exposed to them. If used discreetly they enable one to lead a healthy and stress-free life.

Red:

Red has the longest wavelength and the lowest frequency, making it a strong and vibrant colour. It is the second colour perceived by man after black. Packed with the intensity of fire and blood, it denotes the very primitive and basic instincts and enhances sexuality and willpower. It also affects love, dynamism and energy. Not only does it stimulate the mind but also the body by increasing the blood pressure, respiration and metabolic rate. It has negative implications as well. Prolonged exposure to this colour stresses the mind and causes aggression and antagonism.

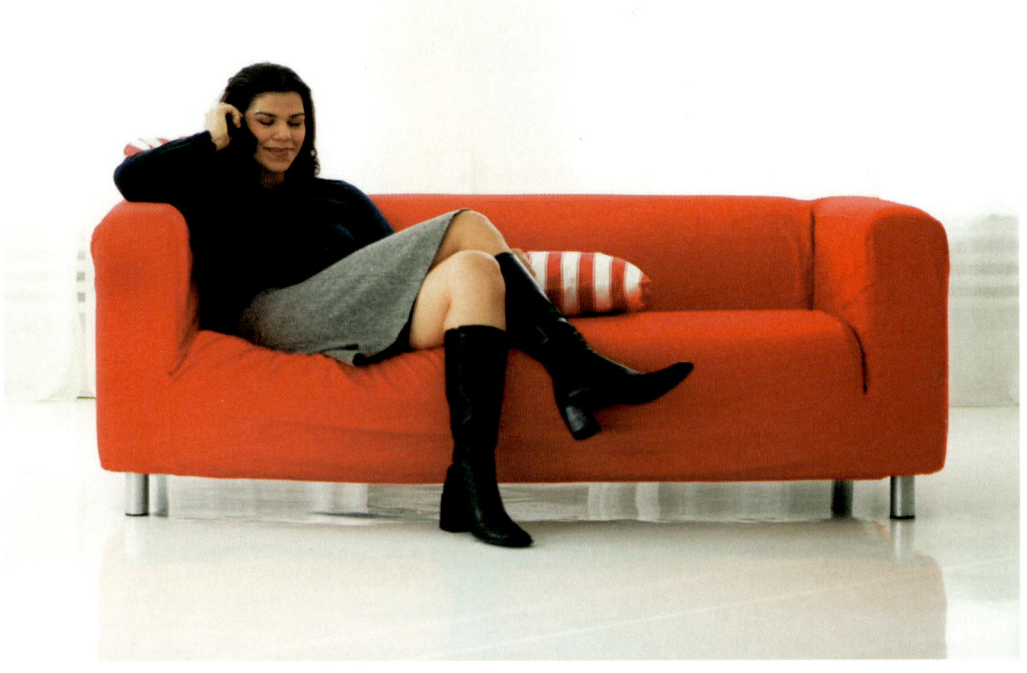

Orange:

This citrus colour is a combination of red and yellow colours. Therefore, it is as warm as the other two colours. It symbolizes liveliness, flamboyance, optimism and is known to be sexually invigorating but it does not arouse passion as the colour red does. It enhances one's creativity as well as imagination at the same time it induces a sense of relaxation. Its negative effect is frivolity, uneasiness and restlessness.

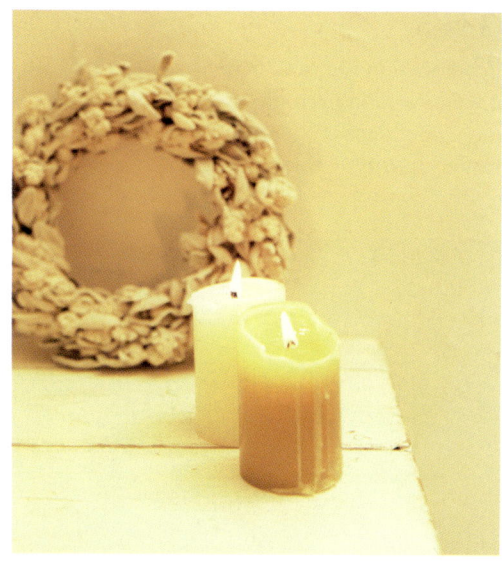

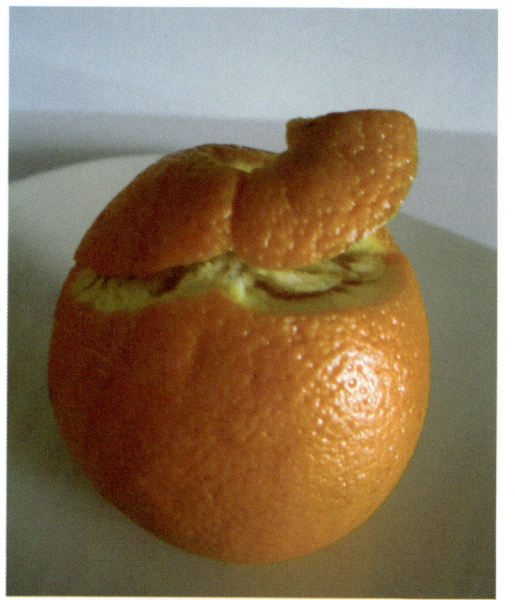

Yellow:

Yellow is reminiscent of sunshine and is just as warm in its character. A colour of wisdom and intelligence, it promotes happiness and a sense of elation. In its highest vibration, it brings out compassion in a person. Yellow is regarded very effective in enhancing concentration levels, in purifying blood and stimulating liver. Its negative impact makes one emotionally vulnerable. Being exposed to this colour in its pure hue for a long period can over stimulate the nerves and cause mental irritation.

Green:

Positioned in the middle of the spectrum, it balances and harmonises. Green is the most abundant colour in nature. It promotes fertility, purity, emotional stability and tranquillity. Green revitalizes the body and is a palliative for a tired mind and body. Negatively, it stands for jealousy and envy. Prolonged exposure to the darker shades of green can cause depression.

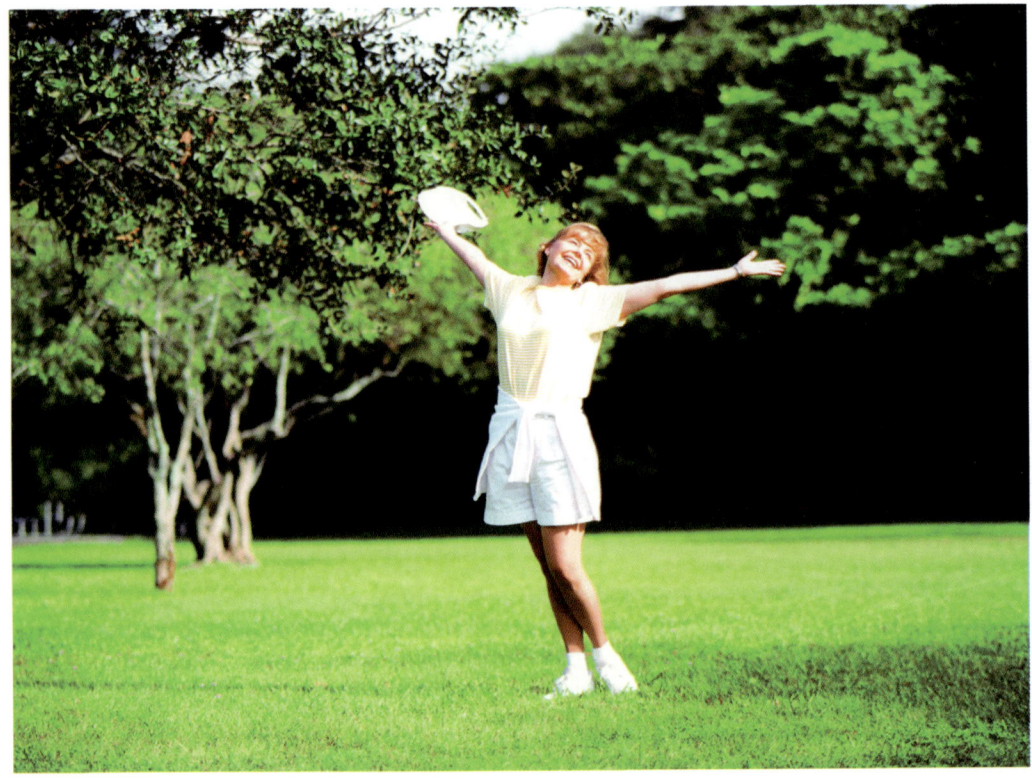

Blue:

This shade of the sky is quite like the expanse above-calm, peaceful and soothing. It is considered restful, known to promote tranquillity and helps to combat insomnia. It denotes correct perception, reliance and trust. Consequently, it lowers body temperature and pulse rate. It suppresses appetite. Prolonged exposure to blue can depress one. Negatively, it denotes a cold and unfriendly attitude.

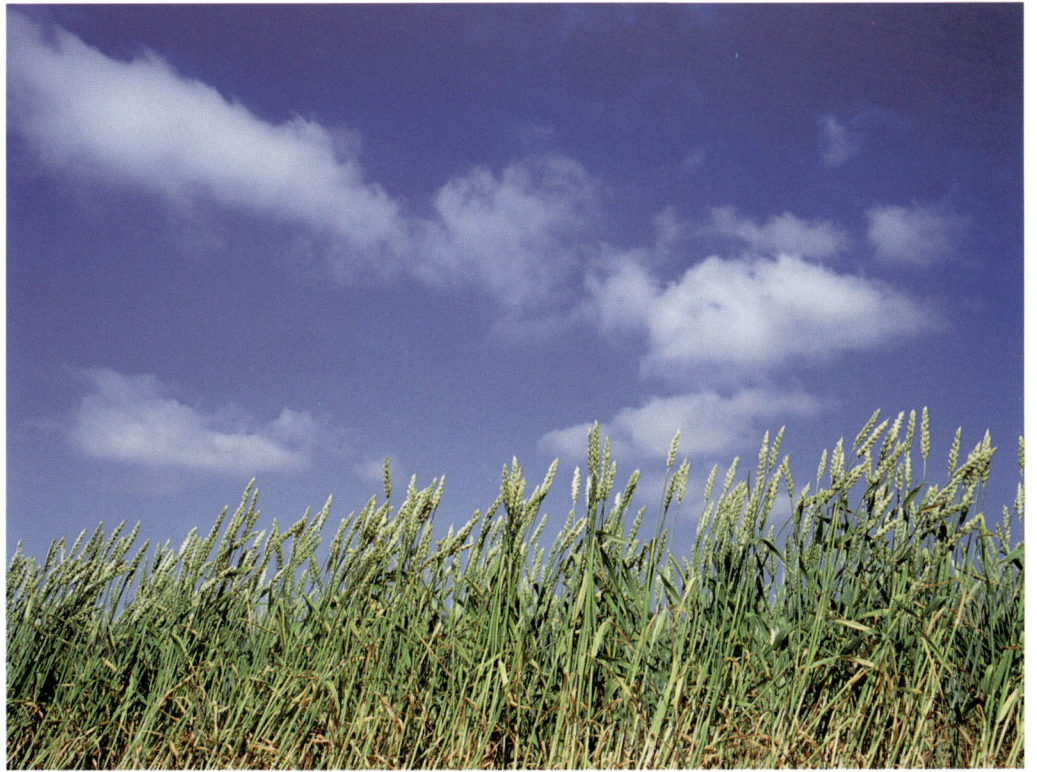

Indigo:

Indigo is a solid colour with no shades or tints. It helps in detoxifying the body, leading to purification. It transforms the mind and soul thereby opening up one's consciousness. It creates a link between the outer and inner being. Indigo enables one to overcome emotional trauma. It is particularly effective when one is weaning away from any form of substance abuse. Its negative aspect denotes an authoritarian attitude and moral rigidity.

Violet:

Violet is a combination of red and blue and so it also combines the energy of red and the tranquillity of blue. It introduces a new world of mysticism and spirituality. Those who delve deep into this colour, are rewarded with psychic manifestations. It enables one to be emotionally strong. It denotes affluence and higher productivity. It reduces menstrual cramps in women. Its negative aspect denotes spiritual conceit and self-indulgence. Prolonged exposure to this colour causes depression.

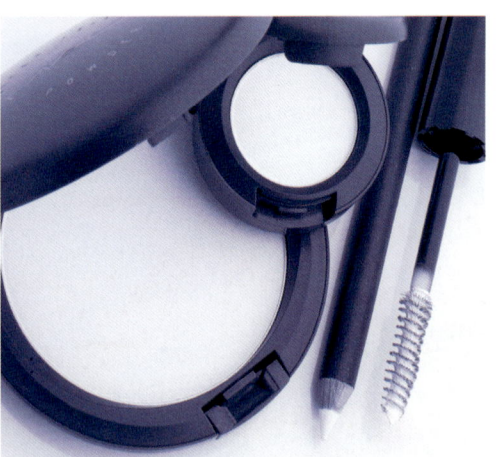

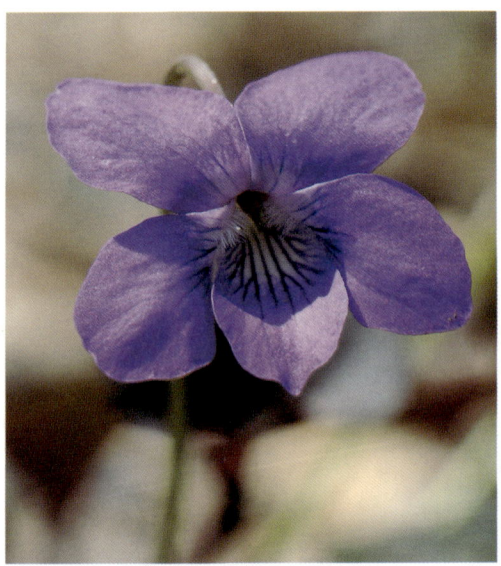

Using This Book

The book has been designed keeping in mind all the stages that a relationship goes through. The book comprises easy-to –comprehend units that deal with all facets of a relationship. It also throws light on which colour is best suited to a particular stage of a relationship. The colours that best enhance a relationship and simple ways of incorporating them in one's life have been mentioned under the following sections:

1. **Interiors:** As colours emanate vibrations that are visually imbibed by the body, they can be effectively incorporated in the interiors of one's home or workplace for therapeutic benefits.

2. **Clothing:** When clothes of a specific colour are worn, the body effectively absorbs the curative properties of that colour. The book suggests simple colour combinations and their unique dualistic effects on one's mind, soul and body.

3. **Food:** The therapeutic value of colours isn't limited to their visual absorption by the body. Fruits and vegetables absorb the light of the cosmos which infuses them with energy that vibrates with the colour of the specific fruit or vegetable. The book suggests consumption of foods and vegetables corresponding to the favourable colour, which enables the body

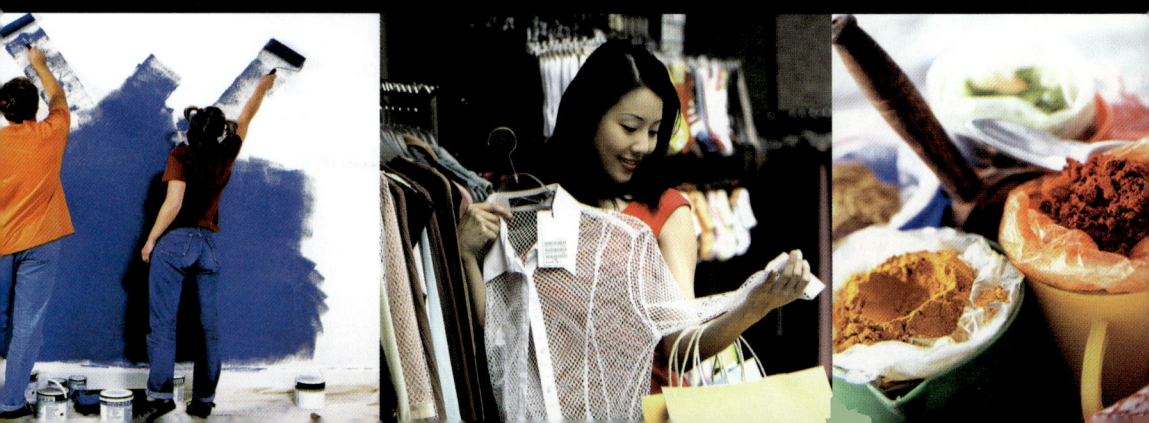

to assimilate the benefits. It also suggests some simple recipes that use the colour-specific fruits and vegetables.

4. **Candles:** Candles not only help in setting the mood for an occasion as is commonly believed but are also, for years, regarded as a compelling medium for channelising the energies of the cosmos and for converting our desires into tangible achievements. The book guides how candles of specific colours can be lit to enable the mind, soul and body to garner energy which facilitates meditative healing.

5. **Fragrances:** Every colour in the spectrum has a corresponding array of fragrances which give the same therapeutic benefits as the colour they are compatible with. This enables a person to benefit from the colours beyond their visual representation. The fragrances mentioned are in the form of perfumes, essential oils and shower gels.

6. **Breathing exercises:** The vital force, breath can be harnessed to absorb the colours of the spectrum without external aids. The book suggests how breathing exercises can help a person unwind and

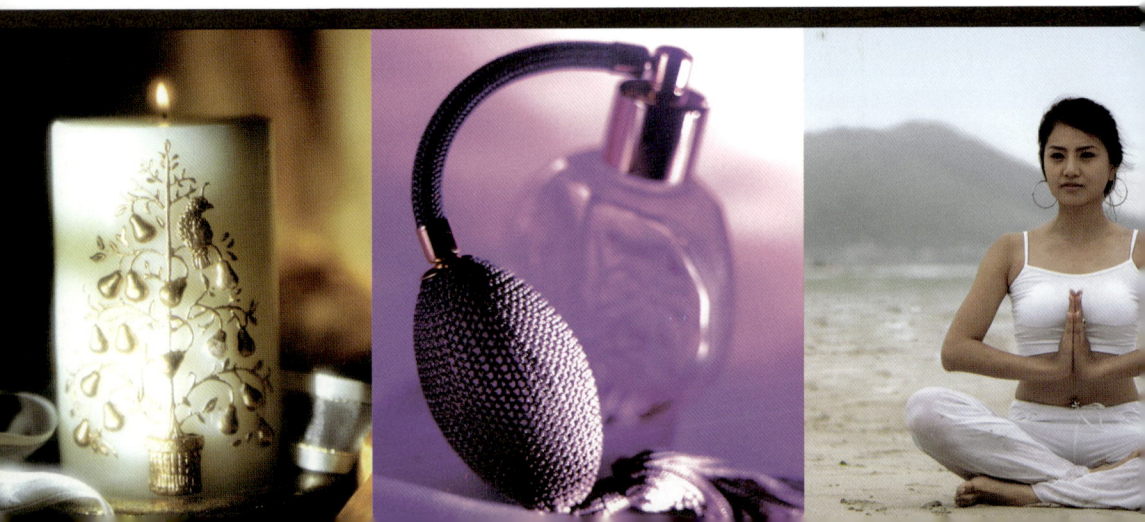

Introducing Colours

simultaneously absorb specific colours through simple visualization techniques.

7. **Gemstones:** The book also touches upon gemstones of specific colours, their unique curative properties, the colour vibrations that they emit and how they can be used as accessories to further assimilate positive energies to harmonise the mind, body and soul.

8. **Music:** Colour and music possess comparable vibrations and frequencies according to Pythagoras. This implies that every colour of the spectrum has its own corresponding musical note. The book offers some musical compositions as examples.

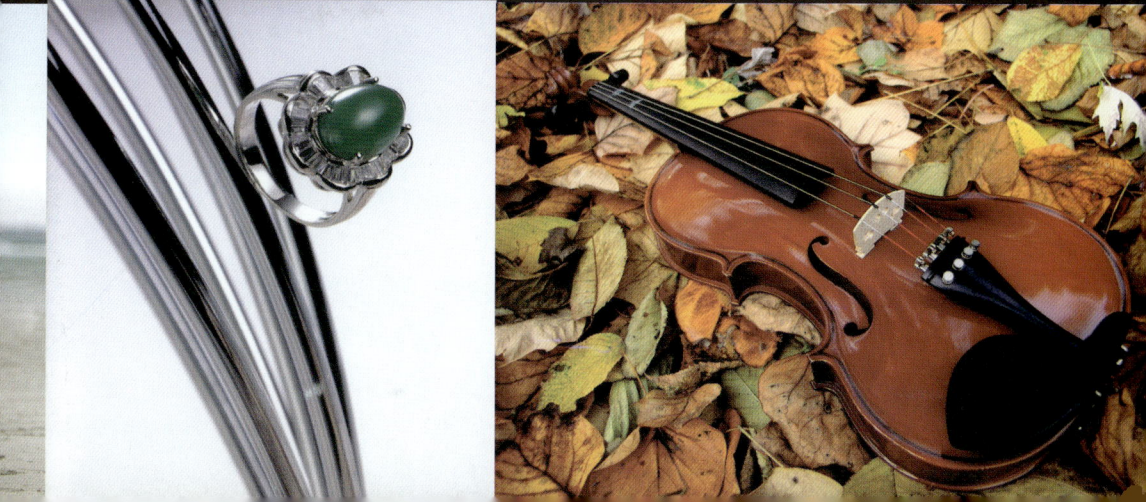

Chapter 2
INTERIORS FOR SINGLES

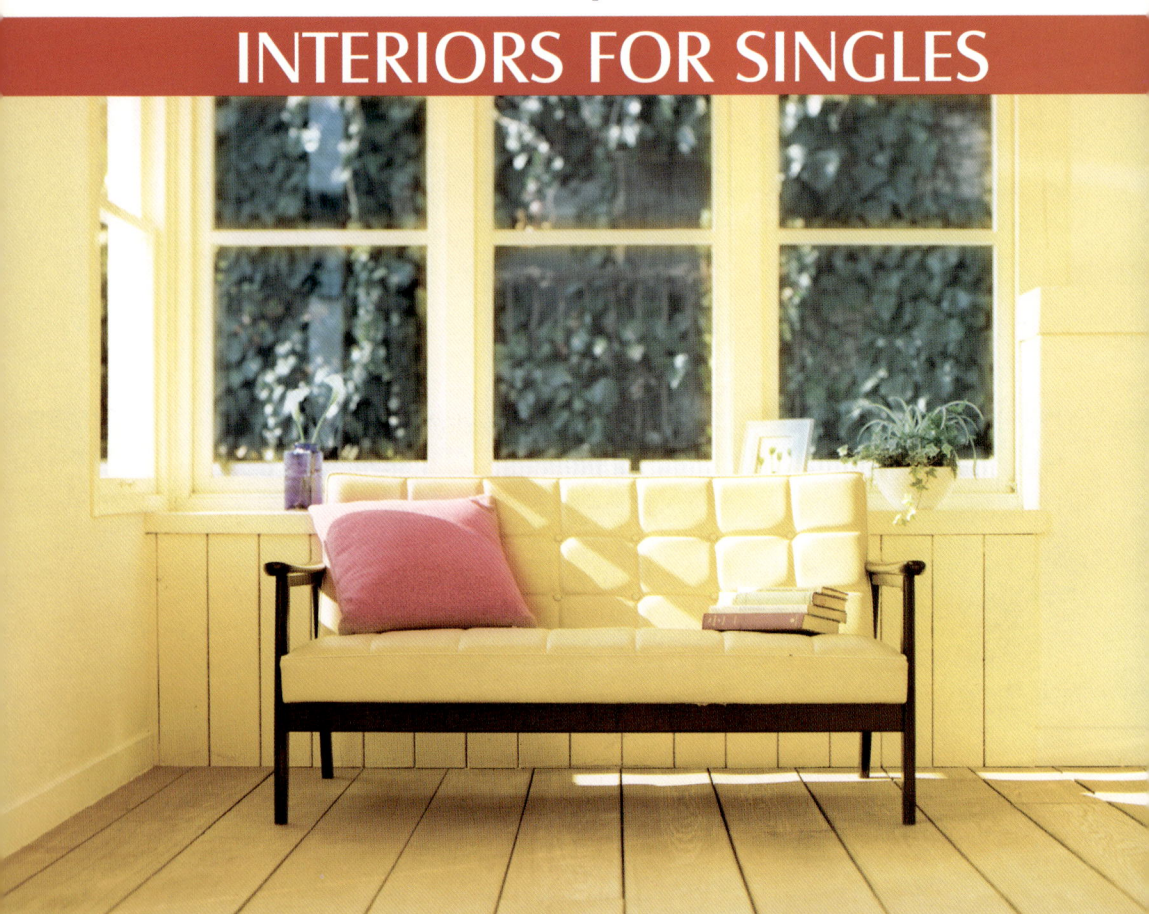

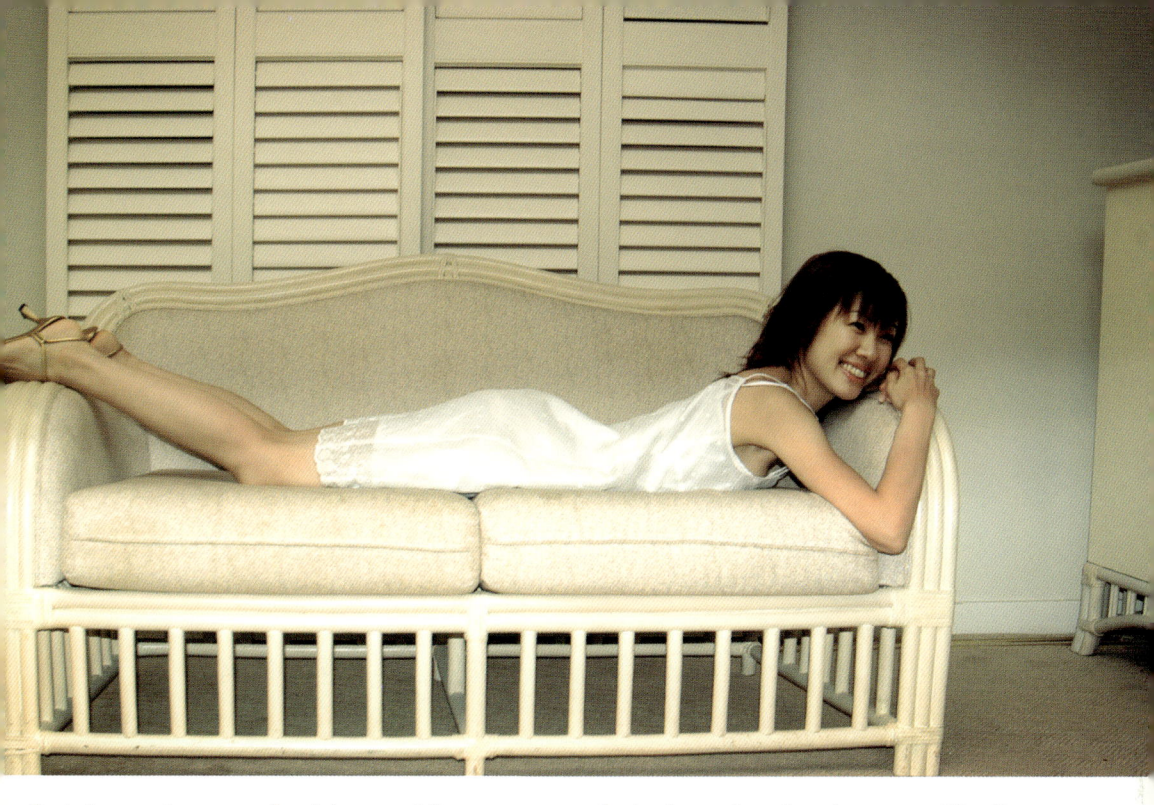

It is imperative to set the right mood for a single person, seeking a loving companion. This starts with the interiors for which the colour tone is essential. Colours subtly but certainly influence behavioural patterns.

Preferably, the colour coordination should be changed for the entire house but if that is not possible, bring changes in that part of the house where the single person spends maximum time while at home. When one is on the look out for a love interest, a friendly warmth would be the right environment. Therefore, soothing colour combinations are most appropriate.

Colours that promote this warmth are different tones of yellow and orange. Orange arouses pleasure and joy. It also enhances creativity which is required by the person to be regarded as open and social.

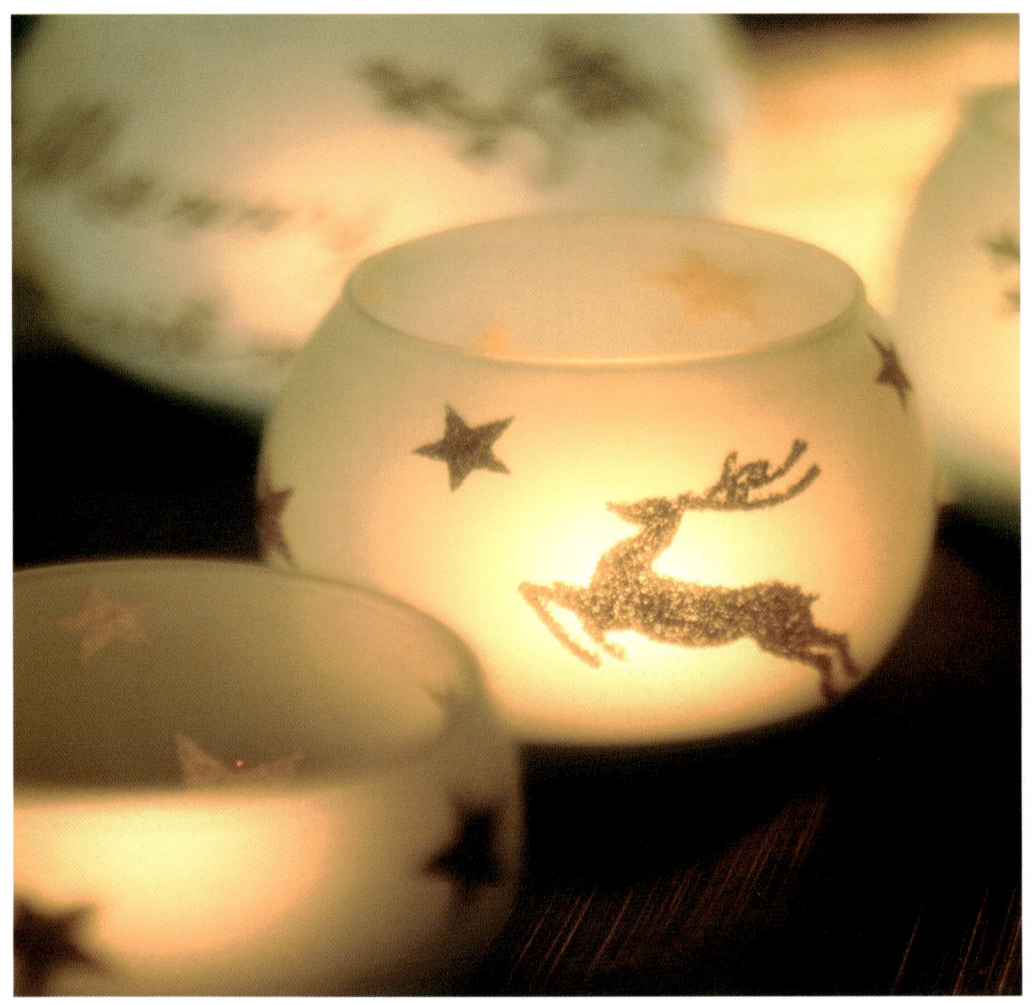

Interiors for Singles

Yellow, on the other hand, conveys buoyant energy and lively movement. It adds to one's vigour, vitality and lends dynamism to the person. Thus, yellow, orange or amber are the best combinations. One must be used as central and the other as a complementary hue.

Shades of brown can be complemented with the principal colour-yellow, for an earthy appeal. This will lend a warm feel to the place, welcoming-enough to attract a loving companion. The use of brown will ensure that the single person is connected to his/her innermost feelings and retains objectivity.

Combining yellow with light pastel shades of purple will have a dual effect. The yellow will keep the person highly motivated, innovative and purple will lend him/her discernment. Such a colour scheme will ensure that the person does not make a hasty or impulsive decision. The experimental ones could try a yellow with green combination. Yellow provides fluidity of movement while green

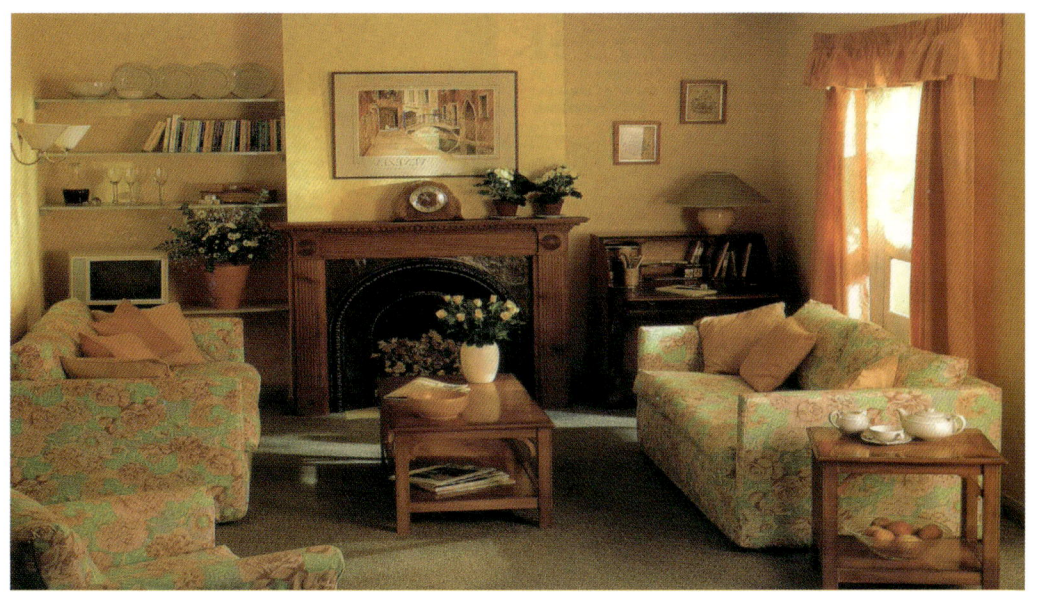

promotes correct judgement and discretion. One mustn't be swept off one's feet while looking for a suitable partner.

If orange is chosen as the principal colour for the interiors, it will promote a sense of elation, pleasure and enthusiasm.

Orange can be combined with various other colours for a binary effect. It can be used with shades of blue which relaxes a person by reducing apprehension and nervousness, natural in such a situation.

Moreover, both men and women like blue so this will not repel either of the genders.

Orange will ensure that the tranquillity of blue does not eliminate joie de vivre. Instead a perfect balance will be established.

The resourcefulness of Orange gets enhanced when combined with slightly reddish hues. Red stimulates the mind and body, making one alert and bringing out one's primal instincts. A word of caution, this combination can easily tire out a person so a calming third colour must be added for a balanced effect. As the third colour, brown is aesthetically more appealing and it also keeps the person level headed.

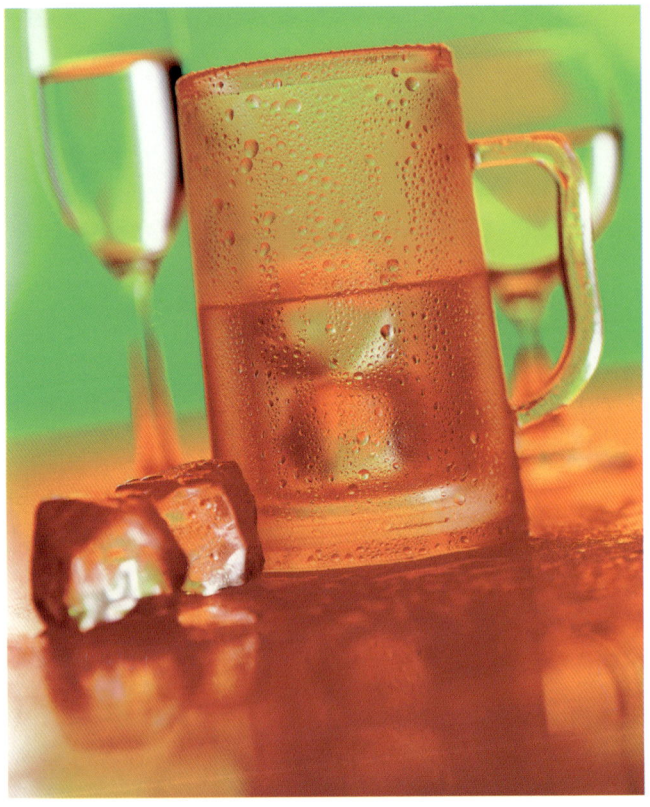

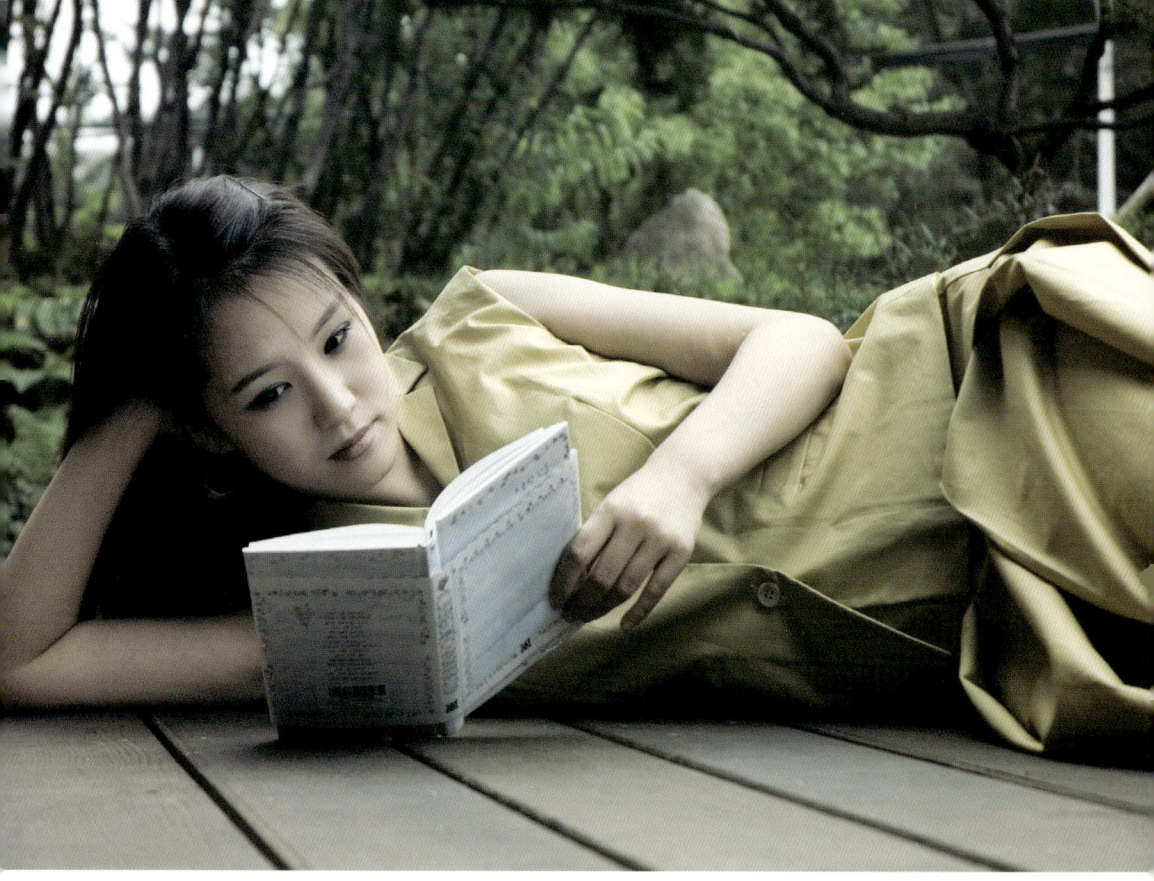

Colours you wear

Once the interiors of the house have been done up using the right colours, the focus needs to shift to clothes. It is rightly said, 'Clothes make the man.' They determine how people perceive you and how you project yourself.

The best colour to wear when looking out for a loving partner is yellow. It is reminiscent

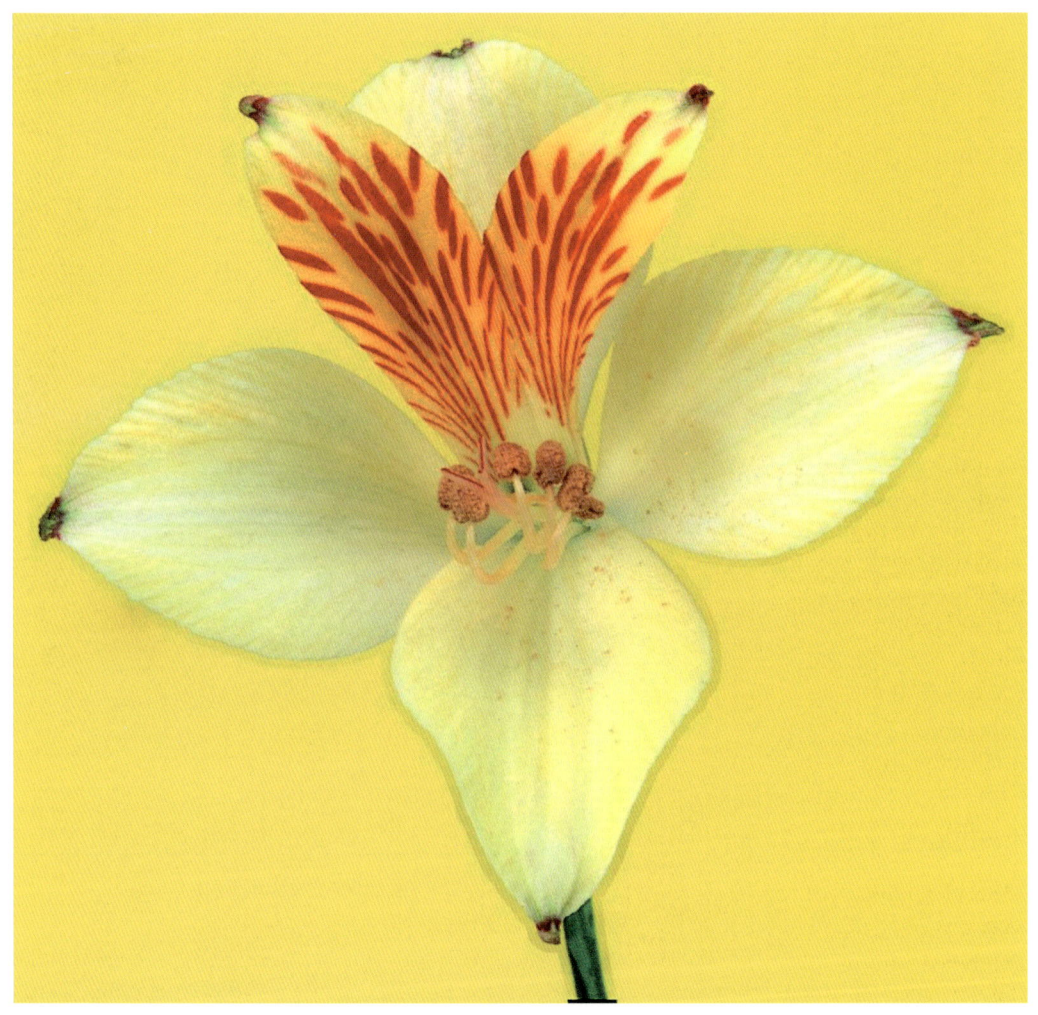

of cheerful sunshine and conveys feelings of mirth and joy, consequently making the one wearing yellow amicable. Yellow is a warm colour which brings forth the warm emotions of a person.

Yellow as a colour has been long associated with imperial status and rank since time immemorial in Asia. Yellow has signified courage for years both in India and Japan, the most needed colour when one is looking for a love interest.

Women find it easy to wear this colour in the form of a dress. They can even accessorise their dress with a gemstone set in gold, a yellow bag or a pair of shoes.

Men, being conservative, would not want to wear this flamboyant colour. They can instead wear yellow undergarments, a tie, or carry a handkerchief.

Yellow can also be combined with the energy-packed orange that would give the ensemble a citrus, summery look. This combination makes the wearer look healthy, by bringing out the brighter skin tones.

Those who prefer classic chic over brassy and glitzy, can opt for the zestful yellow with the elegance of black. Denoting sophistication and power, black conveys a sense of control and discretion without being overpowering

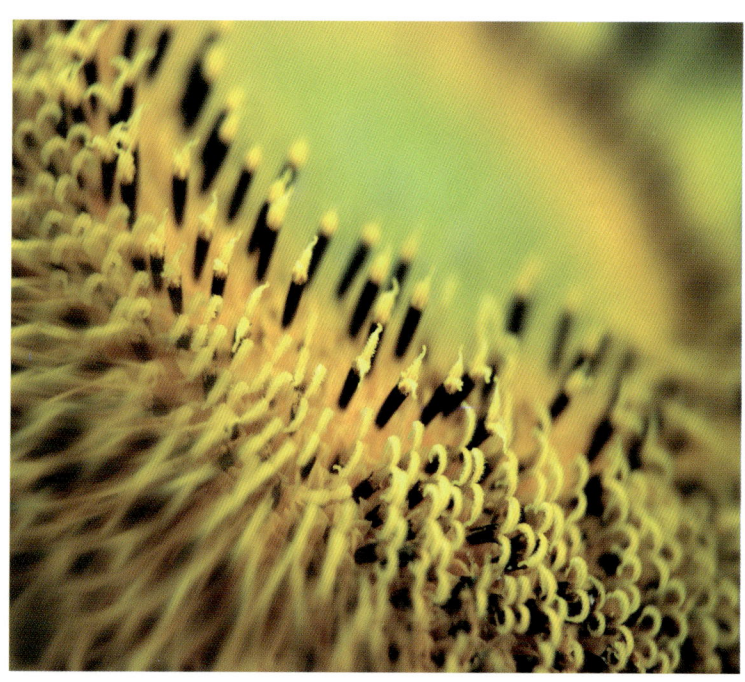

when combined with piquant yellow hues.

There is an eclectic variety of yellow stones to choose from. Topaz fortifies creativity and enhances mental clarity. Yellow diamond is royal in all sense. The yellow Jacinth, considered a stimulant in medieval ages, also guards one from fevers and plague.

There is Amber, in all its various hues like orange, which is scientifically known to protect one from radiations emitted from electronic gadgets. It is good for single men/women as it brings positivism and uplifts the mood.

One, looking for love, has to be noticed first for which no colour is better than orange. It catches the attention immediately. Since this colour denotes enthusiasm and adventure, the one dressed in orange, will be perceived as affable and imaginative.

Orange is the colour choice of the ultra-vibrant and the extrovert. Women, down in the dumps, opt for orange which almost instantaneously uplifts their mood. Women can, not only wear their casual attire in orange,

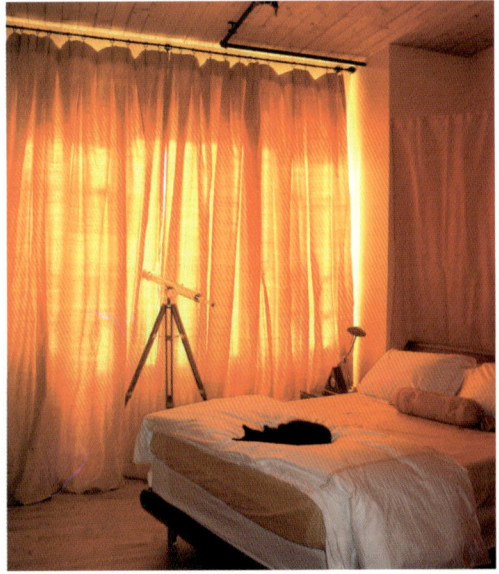

but also have it as the fundamental colour of their night wear.

For the innovative ones, red added to the fiery orange, gives the wearer a high- energy movement, the kind where one can vivaciously waltz through the night without a trace of fatigue.

For an outstanding look which demands a second or even a third glance, orange blends well with white. It fuses the autumnal and the wintry hues without being jarring. White lends simplicity and balance while orange adds the spark of mysticism, both to the apparel as well as to the wearer.

While using gemstones as accessories, one can opt for the dazzling orange calcite, known to enhance feelings of jubilation and optimism. Orange sapphire, alexandrite, carnelian or moss agate are the other options one can choose from.

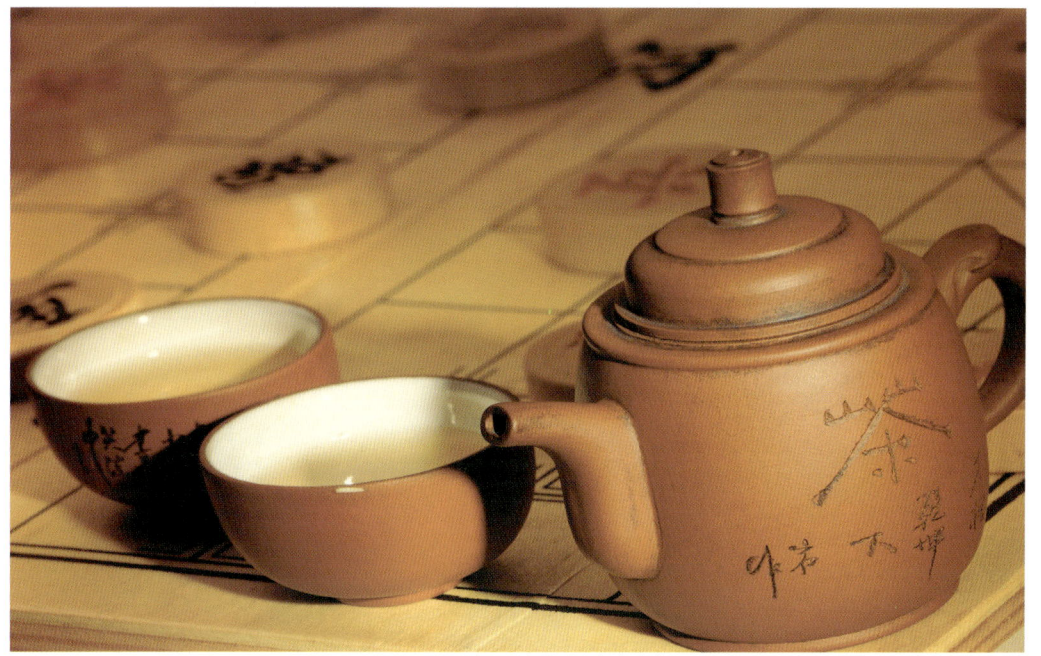

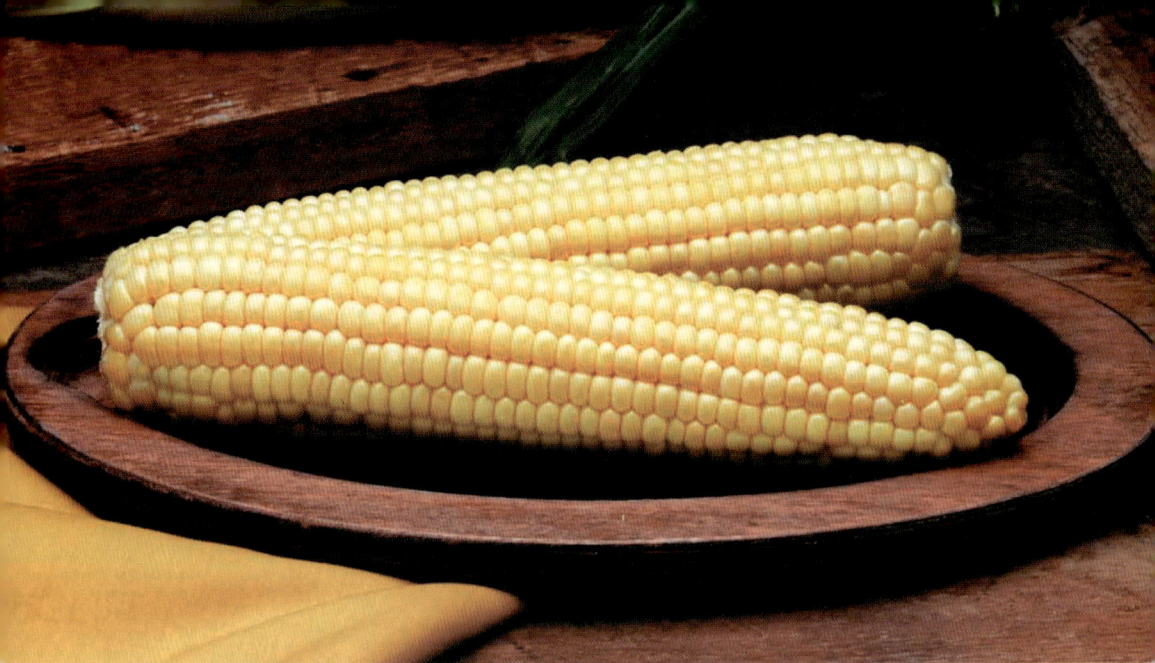

Food for love

Different food items and their colours play a significant role in enhancing one's sex appeal. The colour of the food is absorbed by the body and has the same impact as clothes or interiors. Since yellow benefits the mind and body as a stimulant, by generating muscle energy, bringing clarity and astuteness in perception, it is beneficial to incorporate yellow-coloured food items in one's diet. Fruits like pineapples, bananas, corn, yellow peppers, lemon and grapefruit must be included in the diet by a single person. Here is a simple and quick-to-prepare recipe of a salad:

Papaya and Pineapple salad
Ingredients:

1. 1 pineapple, cut into medium sized pieces
2. 5 orange segments cut into halves
3. 1 large papaya peeled and cut into medium sized pieces

Interiors for Singles

4. Sprinkling of rosemary, coriander and basil
5. 1 teaspoon each of olive oil, lemon juice and orange juice

Method:

Put all the ingredients in a large bowl. Toss well. Refrigerate for ten minutes. Serve cold.

Flowers and candles

When looking for a love interest, one is preparing to blend one's identity with another's. Therefore, preparation must transcend clothing, interiors and cuisine.

This is achieved by incorporating flowers and candles into one's daily fold.

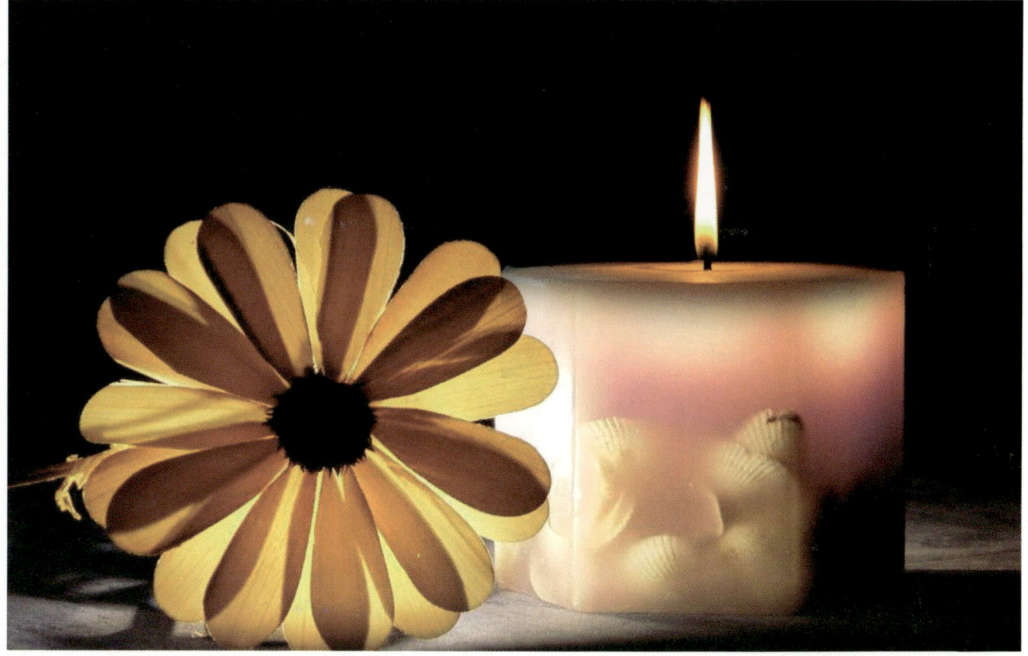

Orange, reminiscent of fire, sets one's mind on fire to search a perfect partner. While making a trip to a florist, look out for ferns, lily of the valley, gardenias or snapdragon for just the right hint of orange.

The more innovative ones may find flowers a bit tame. Such singles must burn yellow candles. This is particularly beneficial to those who are introvert but would like to be forthcoming in their social lives. Candles, not only help in setting the mood for the occasion but are also a powerful medium for harnessing the energies of the cosmos, thereby turning desires into tangible accomplishments.

The candles must be absolutely new and unused since they enhance the effects of the candle ritual.

Burning yellow candles helps in improving one's concentration, boosting energy as well as the creativity quotient. It also makes one's disposition a positive and happy one.

According to candle therapy, burning yellow candles promotes intellect, wisdom and honour.

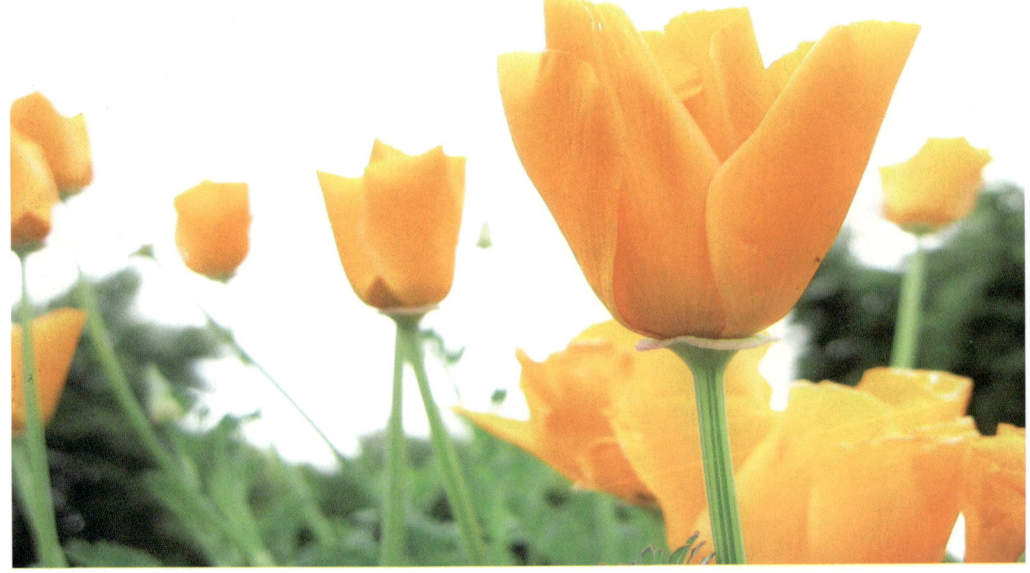

Interiors for Singles

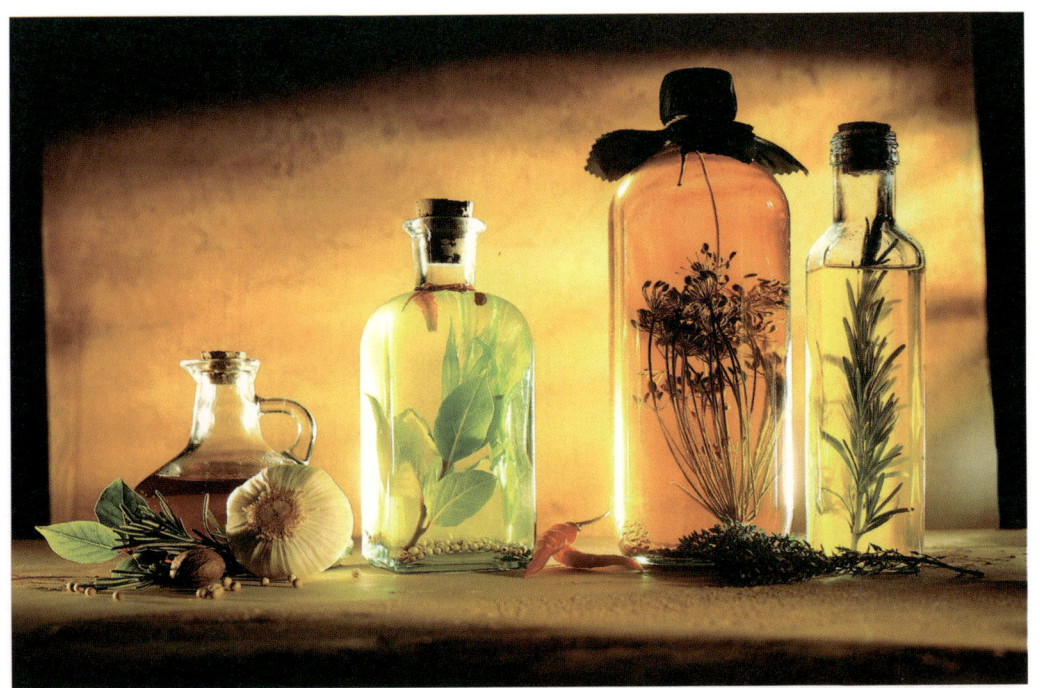

Suitable fragrances

Though the sense of smell is relegated to the last place, certain fragrances evoke strong emotions and often bring back to the mind faint memories.

Every colour in the spectrum has a corresponding fragrance. Since the two colours which work best for single men and women are orange and yellow, accordingly some fragrances suit them more in their purpose.

Jasmine corresponds best with orange. Its fragrance stimulates the mind and makes the person, wearing the perfume, sanguine. The versatile perfume of Lavender will make the

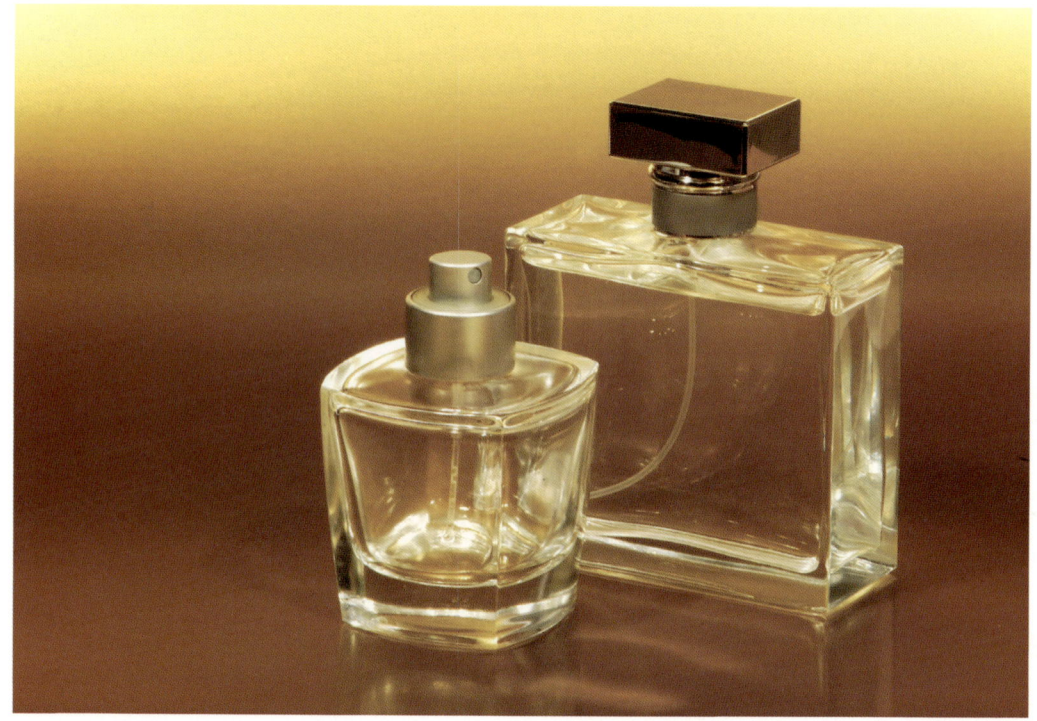

wearer calm and relaxed. Ylang-Ylang is also a good choice. It is not only a delicate oil but also an aphrodisiac. It makes one confident and willing to share one's emotions.

Those who wear yellow have the ever-exotic musk or the essential oils of patchouli to choose from.

People who prefer spicier fragrances can wear clove and vanilla as they both help in calming the mind and balancing one's emotions. Singles, who lack confidence, must choose the oil extracted from the fruits of the Bergamot tree, which adds freshness to one's life and augments poise and confidence.

Colours in nature

Nature has its own way to help man with its myriad colours. In order to benefit from the advantages of yellow, pick a yellow flower and contemplate on it. Look closely, almost meditatively for five minutes to an hour. Slowly as the body absorbs the yellow colour, it will feel empowered physically and mentally.

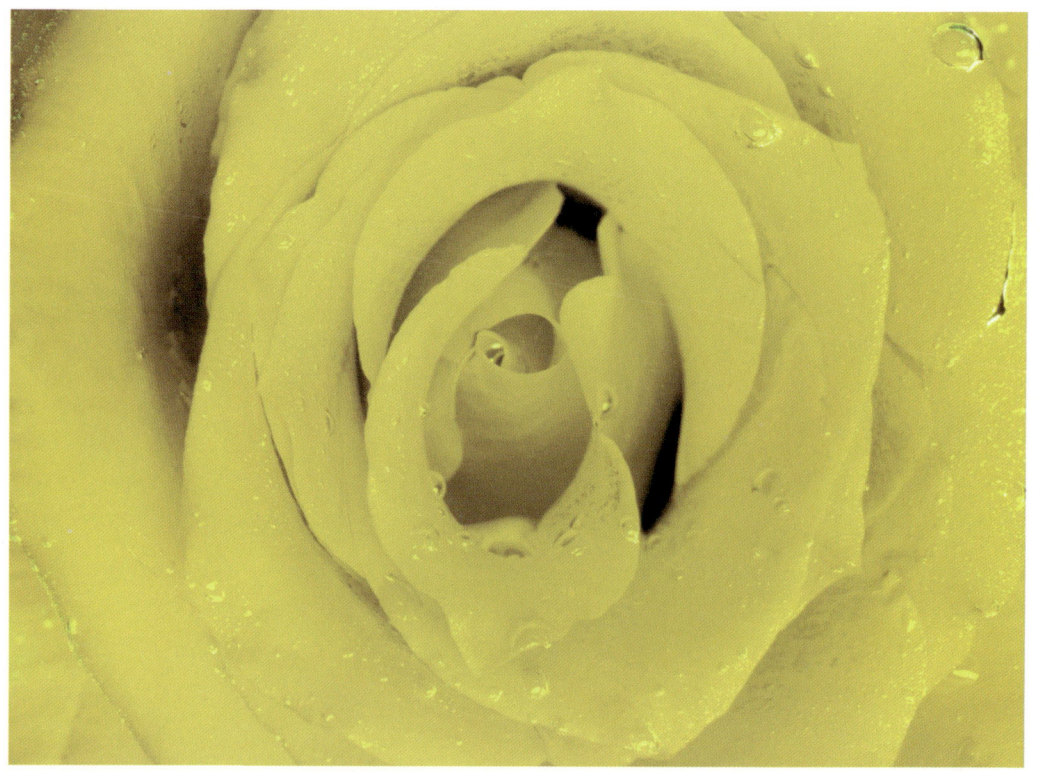

Chapter 3
THE FIRST DATE

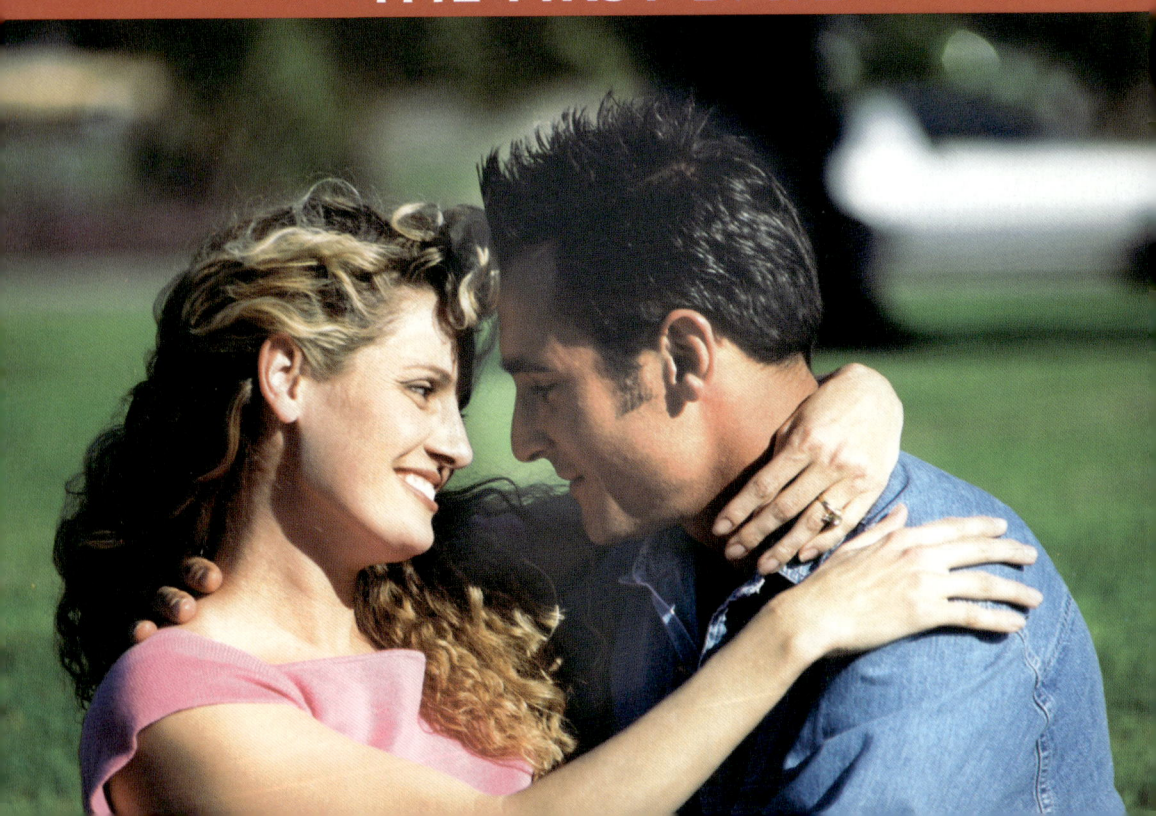

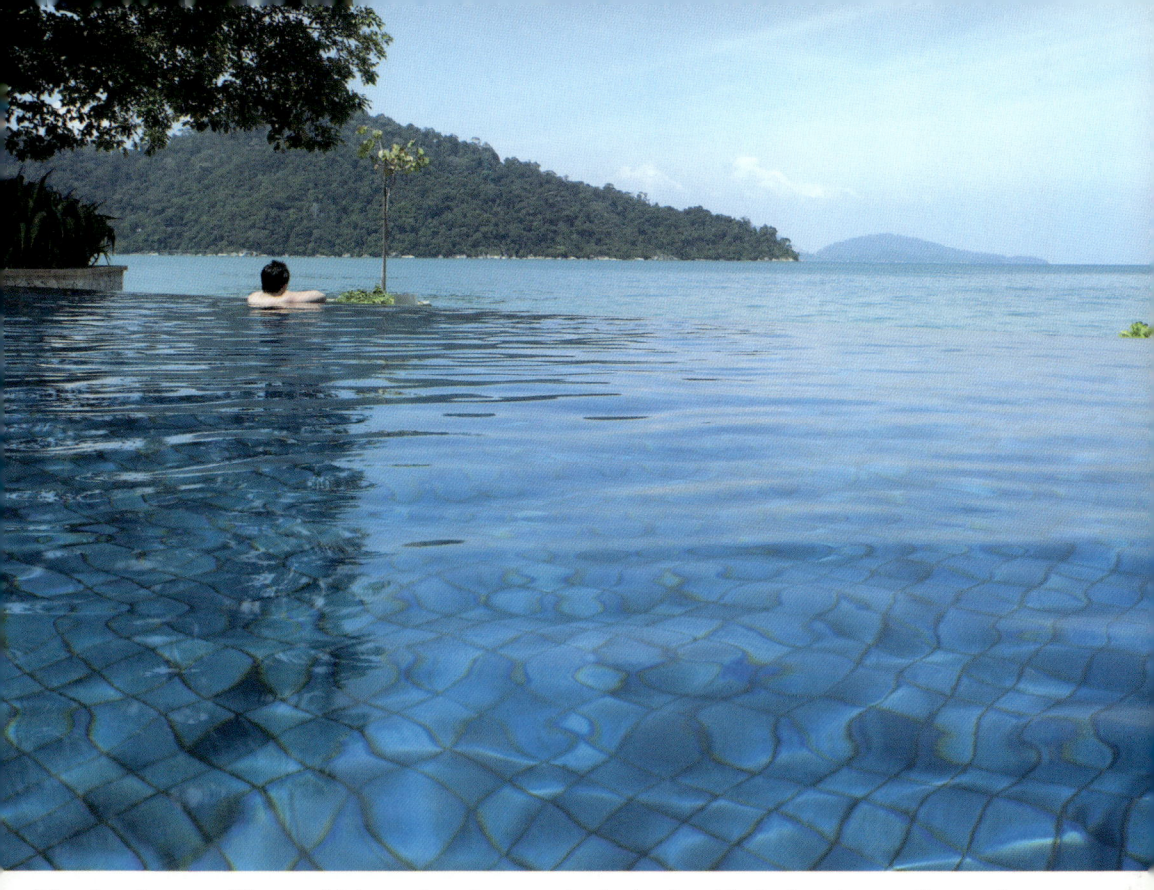

The first date can fill one with lots of anxiety and apprehensions of getting everything right. By making the right choice of colour, the single person can eliminate nervousness and make everything fall into place.

Ideally, one must have a week at one's disposal. Since colours emit coded messages to the brain, begin with the interiors as discussed earlier. Blue, associated with serenity, must be chosen to overcome nervousness. However, too much of blue can result in depression. Use blue along with another colour to avoid the negative effect of using a single colour excessively.

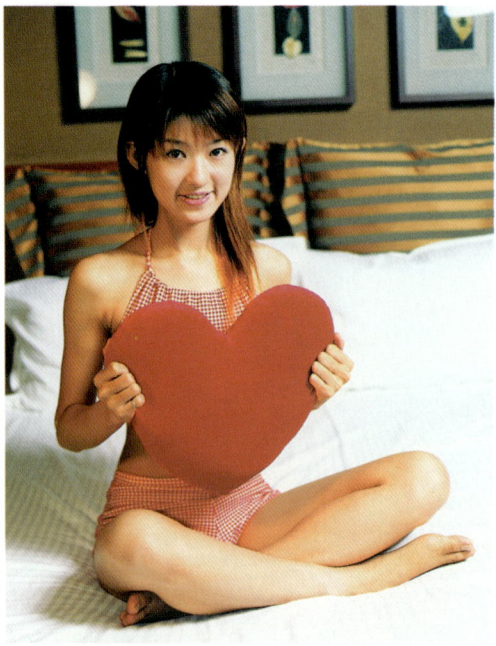

Blue with silver is a classic combination. Silver lends dignity and royalty to the peaceful blue. This combination is good as a dash of silver highlights the blue and the silver enhances the interiors substantially.

Another ideal colour choice for those who feel vulnerable and unsure about initiating contact with the opposite sex, is green. Like blue, this colour is also soothing. Singles for a fondness for green should use olive or sage green for the interiors. These two shades are neither too jarring to the eye nor are they liable to produce any contra effects if used over a long time.

Singles who wish to blend some calm with some zest can use green as a base colour combined with purple.

Green when combined with yellow gives a perfectly poised look to the place. Yellow adds vibrant enthusiasm to a soothing green.

The walls could be blue; the furniture or the linen could be blue. Otherwise, even putting up a blue painting on the wall will have the desired result. The nature lovers can combine blue with tan or brown.

Blue, combined with a rich and intense red, denotes vitality and excitement without making the place too overbearing. Blue will soothe while the red will energise and add verve to the single person.

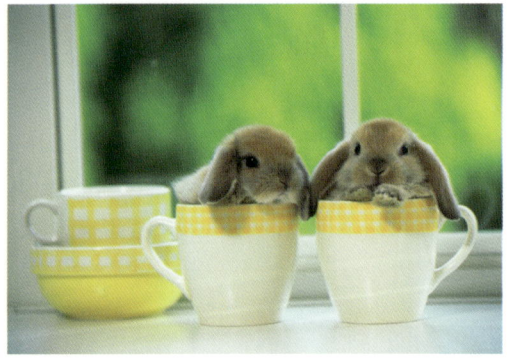

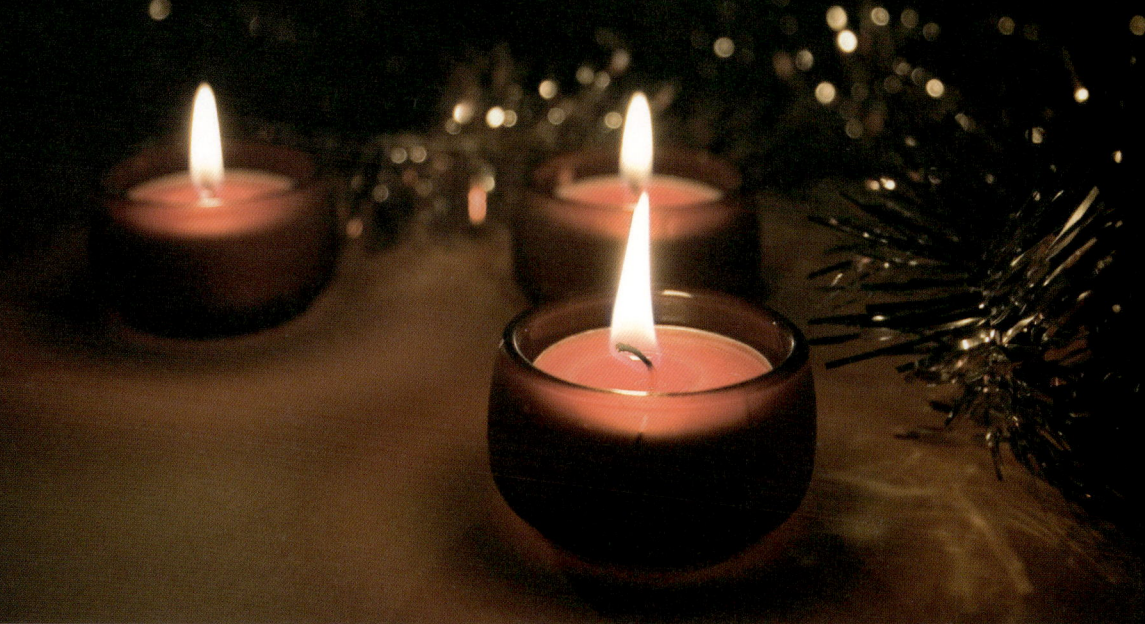

Chartreuse can be paired with magenta by the more innovative. Though this combination is suggestive of high intensity tango, it can tire out one's vision soon. Therefore, discretion in the use of this combination is advised.

One can also purchase candles and give oneself a lift of mood every evening for at least ten minutes so that a week later, the single person heading for a date is relaxed and confident. The colour of a candle for this purpose, is peach- a blend of orange and white. Candle ritual is simple. Start with a new peach-coloured candle. It must be lit for at least 10 minutes for it to affect the mind and body. Light the candle and concentrate on it. It will enhance one's power of concentration and also help the person concentrating on it to imbibe the therapeutic values of peach colour.

The First Date

Attire colours for women:

The most important issue that arises is the attire. Women are bound to be anxious about what to wear on the first date. Before deciding what to wear, it's important to know the location - a formal restaurant, a park, beach or a concert, where the couple intends to meet.

Colour therapy can greatly assist in this process. If a woman wishes to come across as someone with a lot of energy, drive and passion, she must choose a red outfit. Red stirs passion and enlivens the senses. However, it must be kept in mind that red increases blood pressure and respiration rate. So, it is best when toned down by combining it with another shade.

Red with white gives a classic touch. White, a symbol of peace and when combined with the fiery red, creates a soothing balance of power and submission.

Dark crimson can be combined with an equally rich and dark purple for a rich and elegant couture. While crimson symbolizes ardour and passion, purple denotes high spiritual aspirations. Hence, this combination leaves an indelible impact.

The blend of red and black would be best for those inclined towards classic chic. Black denotes sophistication, glamour, lending a mysterious air to the lady in black. It also makes the wearer look thinner Therefore, most women, irrespective of their sizes opt for black.

Pink is another shade which women could choose. It is known as the most feminine colour. Wearing it on the first date is suited as it is a softer, more toned down version of red. According to Feng Shui, pink is the colour of love. It promotes affability in the wearer and also suppresses aggression all around it.

Shocking pink is a brilliant choice for the stylish people who can carry it with panache. It's high concentration of red makes the wearer come across as a vivacious and engaging person to be with. This colour also ensures that the woman wearing it, feels feminine, outgoing and more in control of herself.

However, too much pink can drain the body. This can be avoided by combining it with green for a well defined style statement. Moreover, this combines compassion and warmth of pink with the youthful zest of vibrant green.

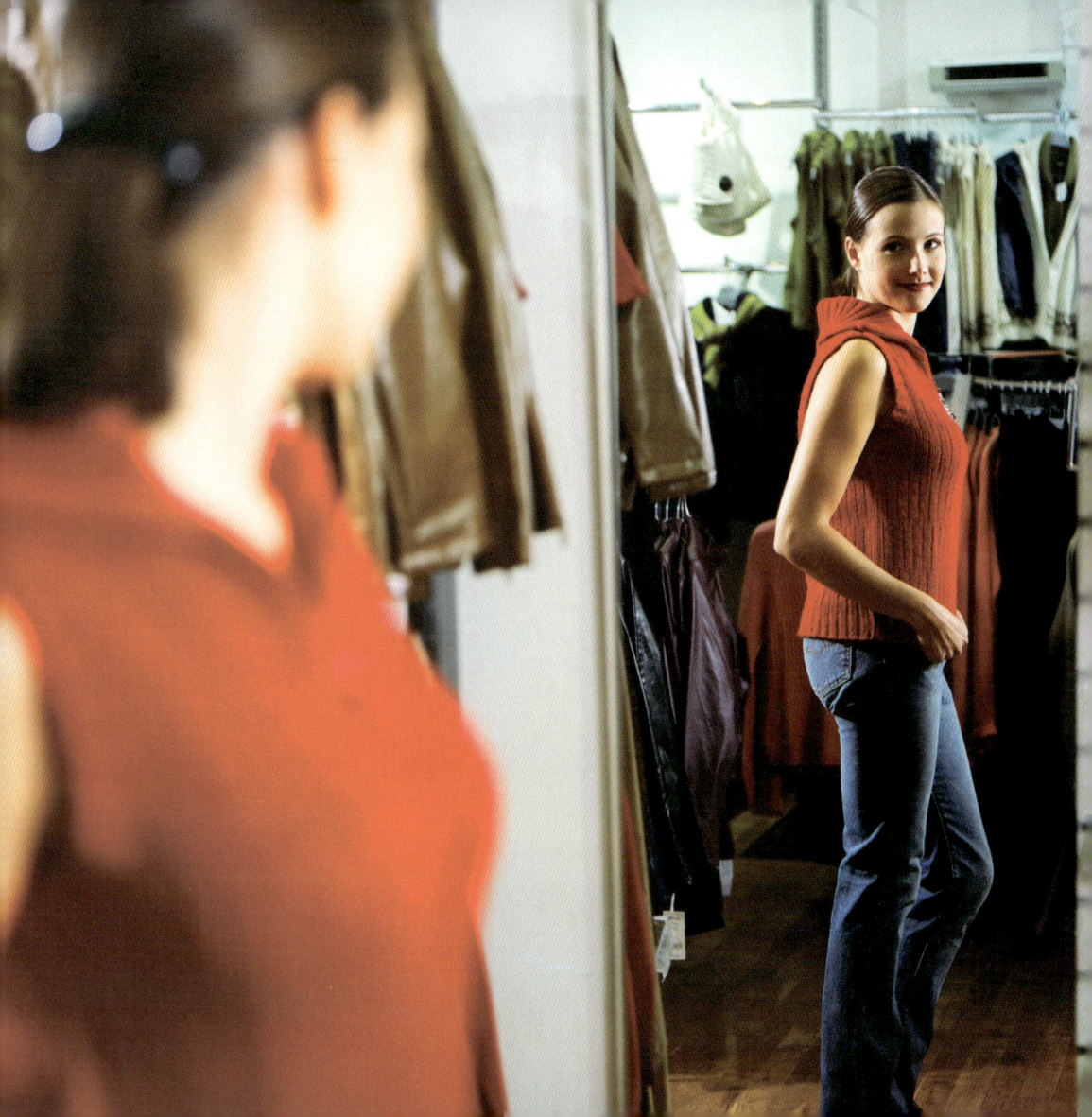

Combining pink with steel grey, lends the wearer sophistication and poise. Grey is regarded as emotionally neutral and denotes dignity and solemnity. Pink adds a dimension of affection and conviviality to it. Grey is also associated with wisdom and maturity. Therefore, those who would like to be taken seriously, no matter what be the occasion, must opt for grey. Pink and grey pin stripes work wonders for those women who wish to appear taller than their actual height.

Another good combination is of peppy pink with blue for a peppy and piquant look. Blue makes a person feel peaceful while pink adds an element of cheer not just to the attire but also to the mental makeup of the person.

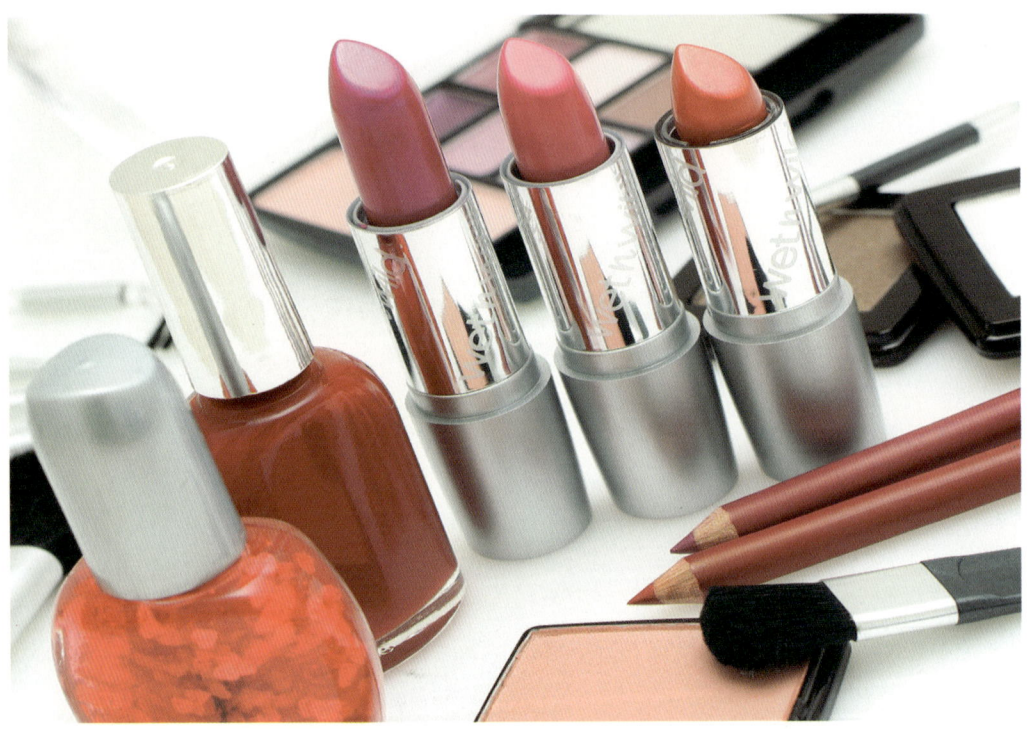

The Perfect lip colour:

The lip colour plays a very significant role as the woman's face is likely to attract all attention. Her face is a canvas of expression in which her lips convey a lot.

The lip colour must be coordinated with the colour of the attire as well as one's skin tone. The ideal lip colour for the first date is red. Being sensually provocative, it is directly related to passion. However, all reds do not suit all skin tones.

For people with warm skin tones with yellow undertones, brown- based reds suit best. An array of reds ranging from warm reds to tawny reds enhance other skin tones.

Girls with cool skin tones should opt for the pink tones of red that include berry and brick reds. They can also choose from plum and blue tones of red, which also make the teeth look pearly white.

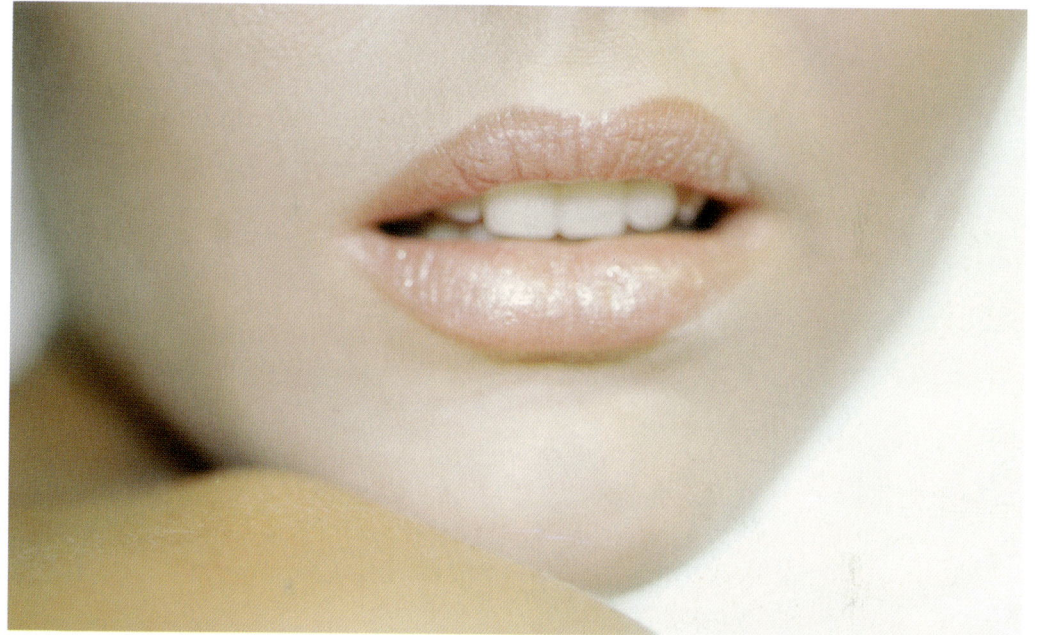

After the girl has decided upon the dress, she should focus on the fragrance. This must be in accordance with one's essential nature.

Ideal Fragrances:

The ideal fragrance for a woman on her first date is one which complements the colours red or pink and in such cases, the forerunner is the scent of strawberries. The scent of strawberries is a good choice as it is suggestive of spring time. It makes one more energetic and positive. One can use strawberry-scented face wash and a moisturizer and not a perfume.

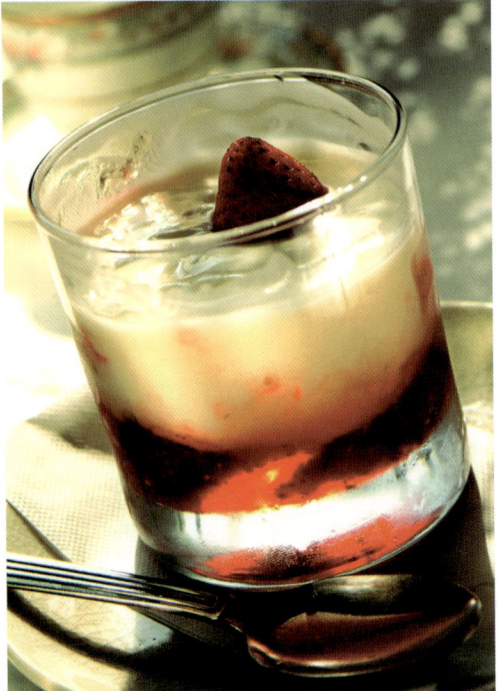

Another fragrance that corresponds to the pink colour is that of the ever-exotic Ylang-Ylang. This fragrance uplifts one's mood and is used as a relaxant. There are a multitude of perfumes available that carry a hint of Ylang-Ylang and a dash of it is all that is needed to make the first date memorable.

Some other equally effective fragrances that carry the positive effects of pink are jasmine, apricot, lavender and sandalwood.

Attire colours for Men

Red, which grabs attention, must be combined with softer shades like somber blue. A solid blue shirt will perfectly offset a bright, vivacious red tie. It has been scientifically proved that blue-based reds attract women more than any other shade. Steel grey perfectly complements and tones down red and so, is a good choice for the men folk. A red and grey striped shirt lends so much charisma and sophistication that a woman is barely able to keep her eyes off him.

Every man may not like to be the centre of attraction. The softer shade of orange is an

The First Date

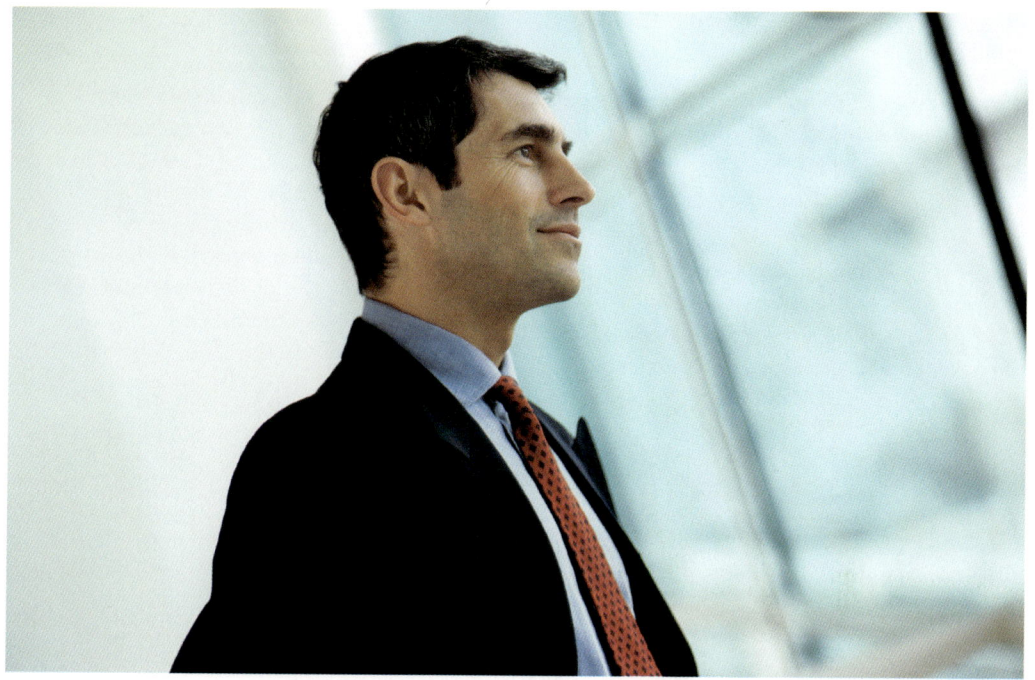

ideal choice for such men. It combines the passion and intensity of red with the liveliness of yellow. It is easy on the eye and men clad in orange are regarded as high – spirited and fun loving.

Orange with black gives a restrained and sophisticated look. This dual colour combination exudes reliability. Orange combined with earthy brown makes a person more approachable, trustworthy, modest and friendly. Orange with a hint of green can be tried by the innovative ones.

After attire, the next important issue (for the first date) is a suitable fragrance. One must exude a sexy tantalizing effect. Colognes with cinnamon, rose, musk, patchouli or cedar are great choices for they correspond to the erotic red.

Flowers for the first date:

Men, as a rule, should never meet their date without sweet-smelling flowers. Both orange and pink flowers work best for the first date. Red flowers can be left for another intense occasion on a later date.

The colour of a flower denotes a particular emotion. Different flowers convey different messages. Therefore, when a particular flower of a specific colour is presented, it conveys the purpose and the feelings of the person presenting it.

Presenting a bouquet of orange flowers, conveys that the person prefers a warm and friendly relationship to a sizzling and intense one. Orange carnations speak of a desire for love and a commitment of fidelity. Lily of the Valley denotes that the one presenting the flowers has the strength to harbour and nurture true love. Ferns convey a kind heart while Gardenias denote cheerfulness, jollity and joy in a relationship.

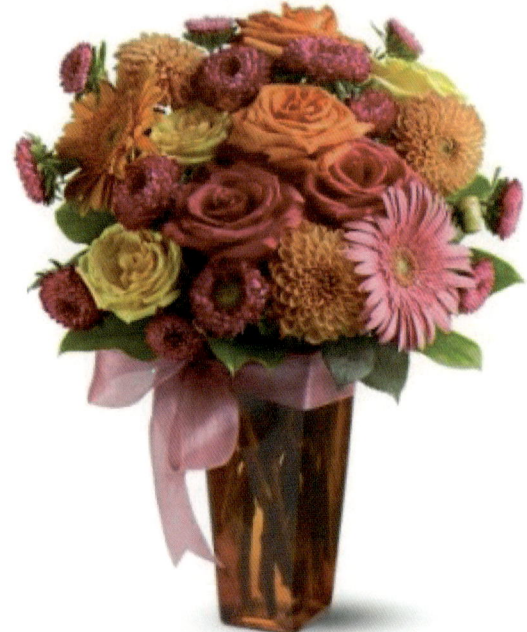

The First Date and Dinner:

Statistically speaking, most couples choose to dine out on their first date. It is essential that the date comes to an end with both enjoying the evening and wishing to meet again.

Some colours can help in making the dinner a truly memorable one.

An eatery with vibrant colours like red and yellow on its walls will lend wisdom, joviality and warmth to the occasion.

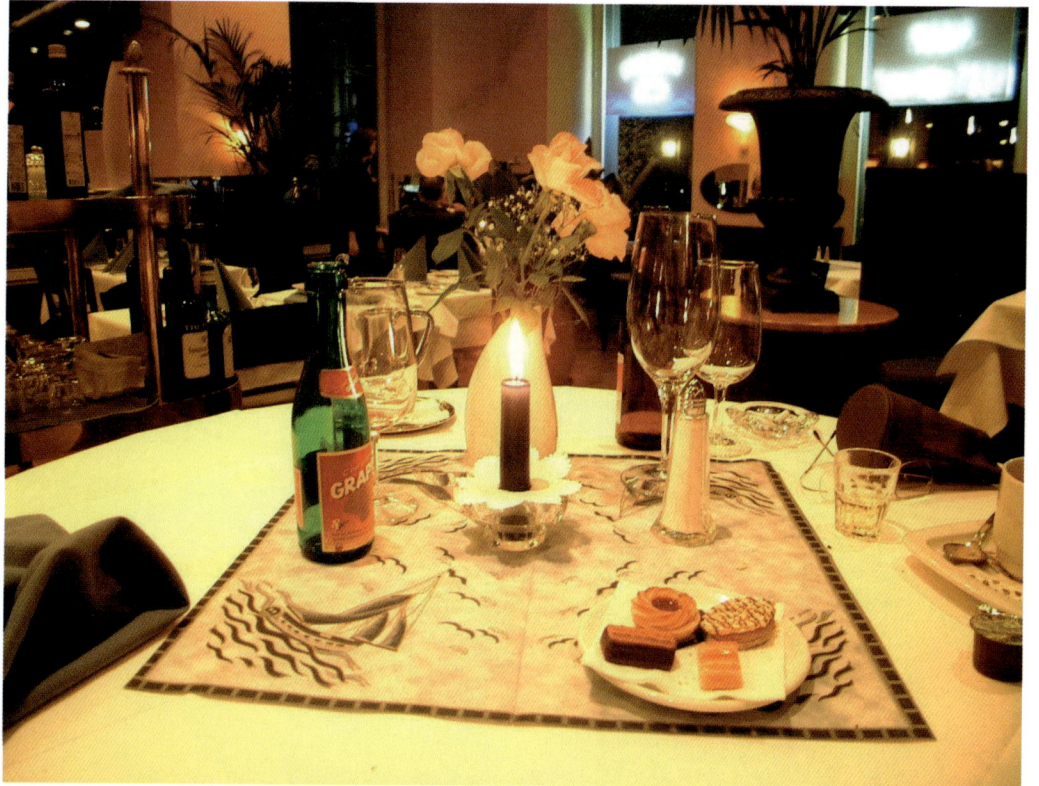

Chapter 4
KNOW YOUR PARTNER THROUGH HIS FAVOURITE COLOURS

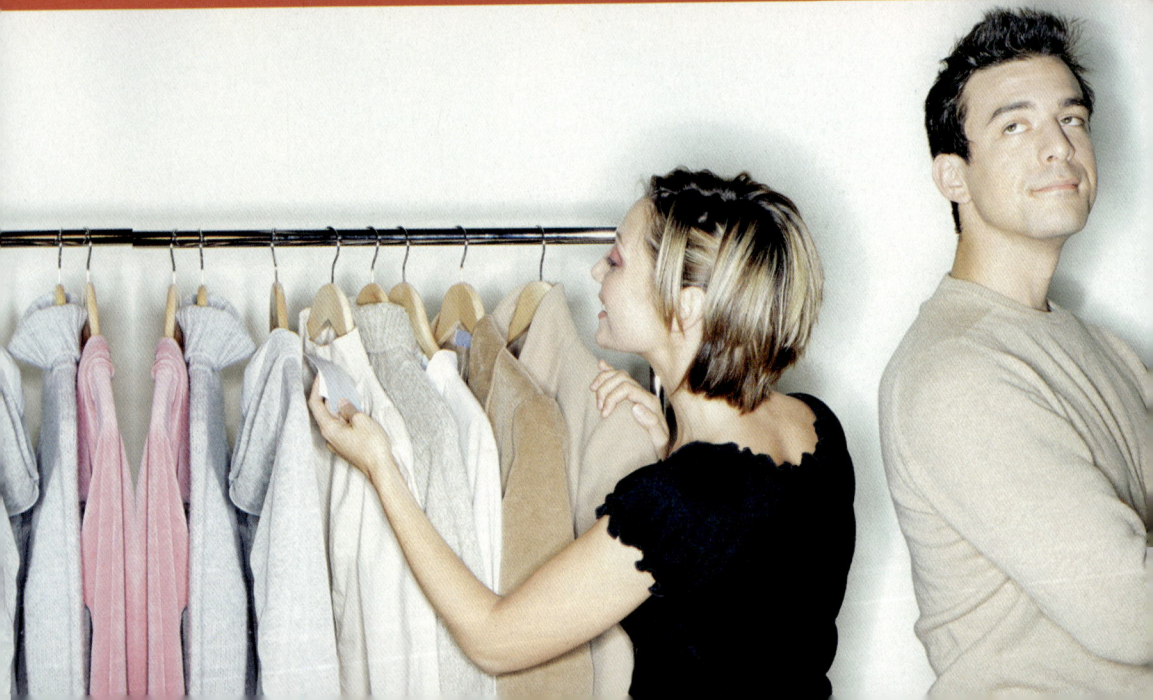

Know Your Partner Through His Favourite Colours

Human behaviour is an enigma and multi dimensional. Yet, when it comes to a loving and fulfilling relationship, one desires to know the partner intimately.

One easy and effective way to know your partner is simply to know his/her colour preferences. Knowing the partner's favourite colour would reveal a lot more about his personality than ten dates put together.

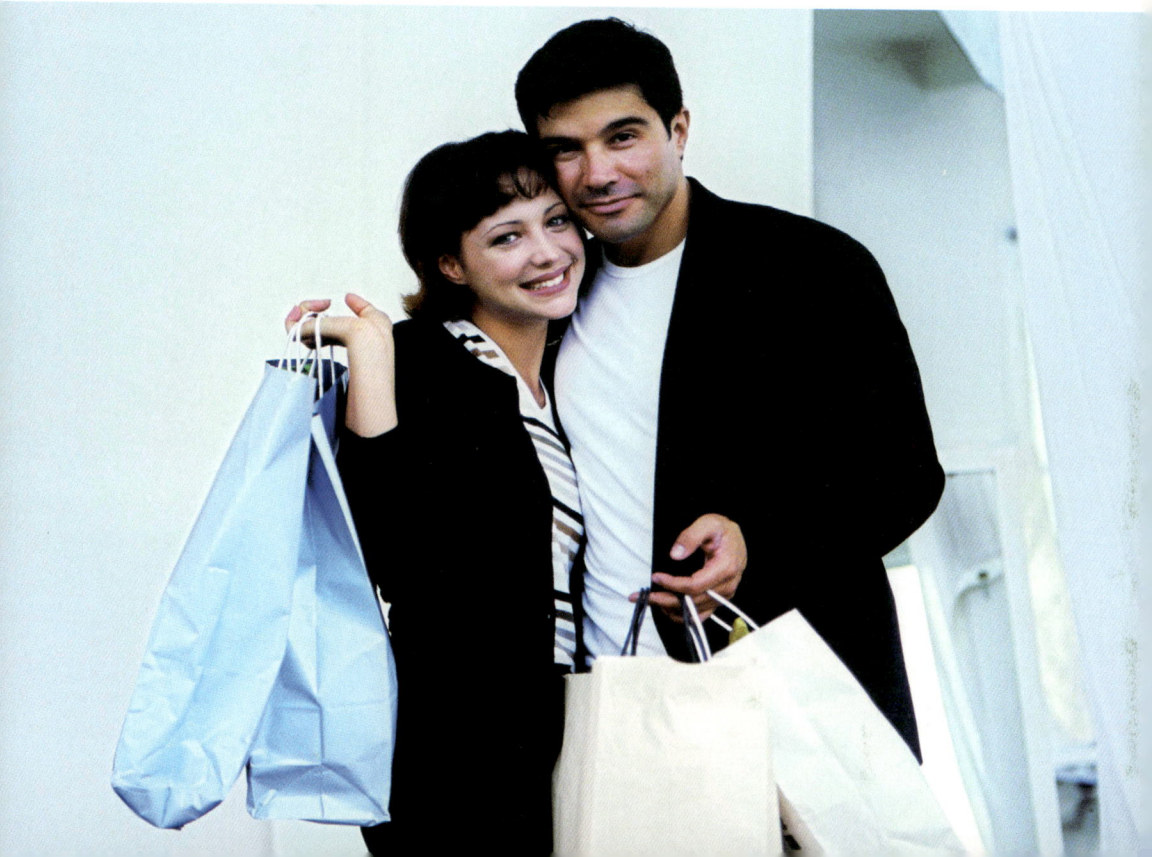

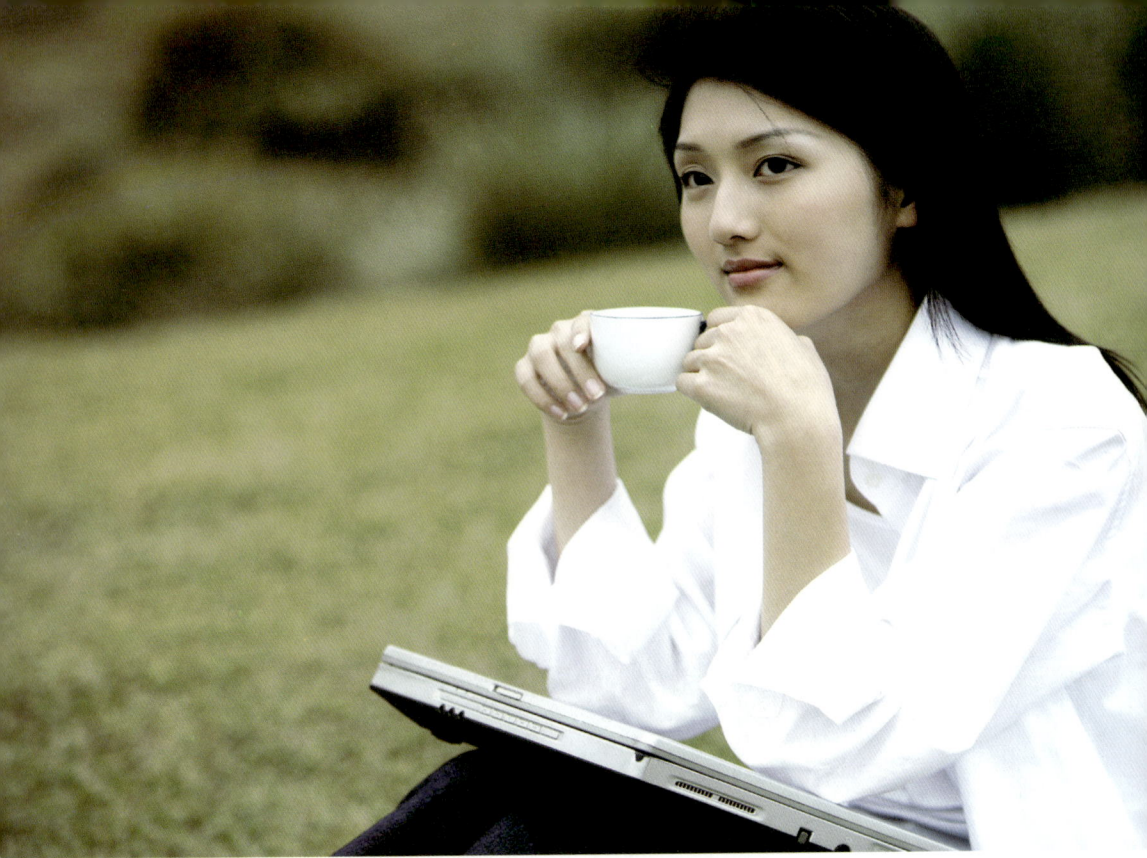

White:

This colour symbolises purity and innocence, which is why brides in western countries wear white. A white bridal gown suggests flawlessness and youth.

People who prefer white, desire perfection and orderliness. It may also indicate that the person wishes to bring about a certain change in his/her life or that he/she is hoping to recall lost glory and freshness.

People who love white are easy going and cheerful. They are open to suggestions and are willing to change which is exactly what a relationship needs. White also stands for truth and therefore symbolises a person's desire to lead a simple and honest life.

Purple:

A person with a passion for purple is individualistic with strong opinions. He harbours the desire to be unique and different from the rest. One who loves purple has the qualities of a leader and invariably stands out from the crowd.

These people are witty and keen observers of things that might skip others' notice. They are adventurous and spontaneous. A person who prefers purple to other colours is likely to be temperamental even in situations which go against him/her. He/she becomes excessively garrulous and argumentative when under stress. When misunderstood, such people detach themselves and become loners and slightly sardonic.

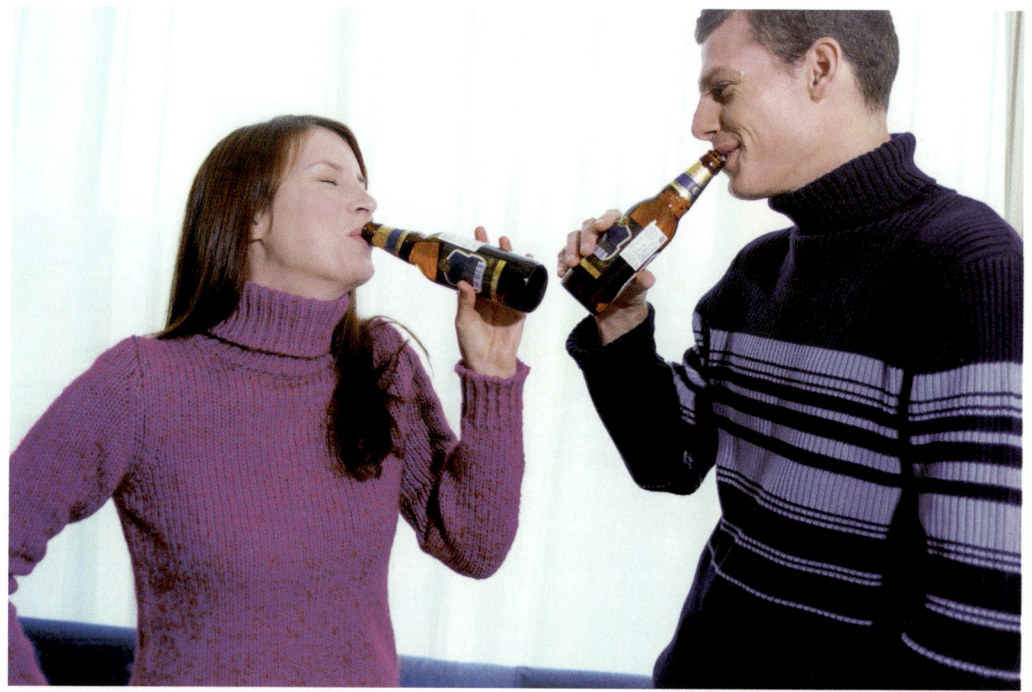

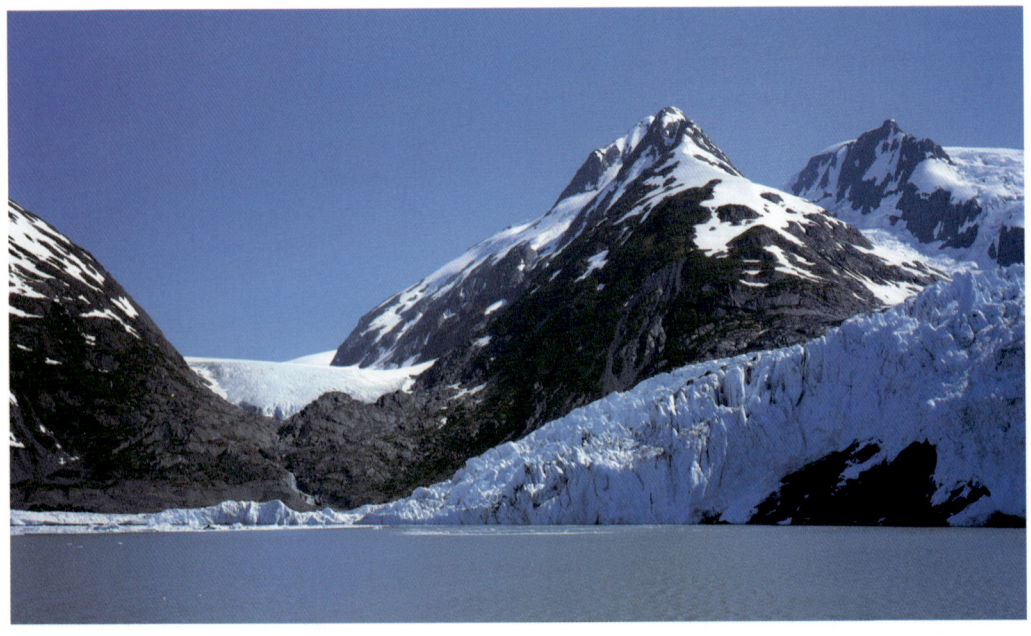

Blue:

Blue, traditionally associated with the sky and the sea denotes peace and stillness. People who like blue the most, are inclined to enjoying tranquillity and have a laid back approach to life. This allows them the time to appreciate life and nature. Such people are temperamentally introspective, solicitous and concerned about others' feelings, making them very considerate people.

The lovers of blue are great conversationalists who freely express their views. They are serene, sober, meditative dreamers, who seldom act to realize their dreams. However, when truly determined, they can face all odds to accomplish their mission. They love harmony, give importance to love, emotions and therefore ostentation puts them on guard. When under stress, they withdraw to a peaceful environment. They are the most dependable friends and most loyal lovers.

Green:

Green symbolises serenity, abundance and renewal. Like the lovers of blue, people who prefer green to other colours are gentle, mild and love peace and tranquillity.

A typical trait of people who love the colour green is that they are the pillars of the community and hold the greater good of humanity above selfish gains and benefits. They are moralistic people who consider sincerity and trust worthiness to be of utmost importance in their own lives and expect the same from other people.

Green lovers are also art lovers and appreciate the finer, more beautiful things of life. In

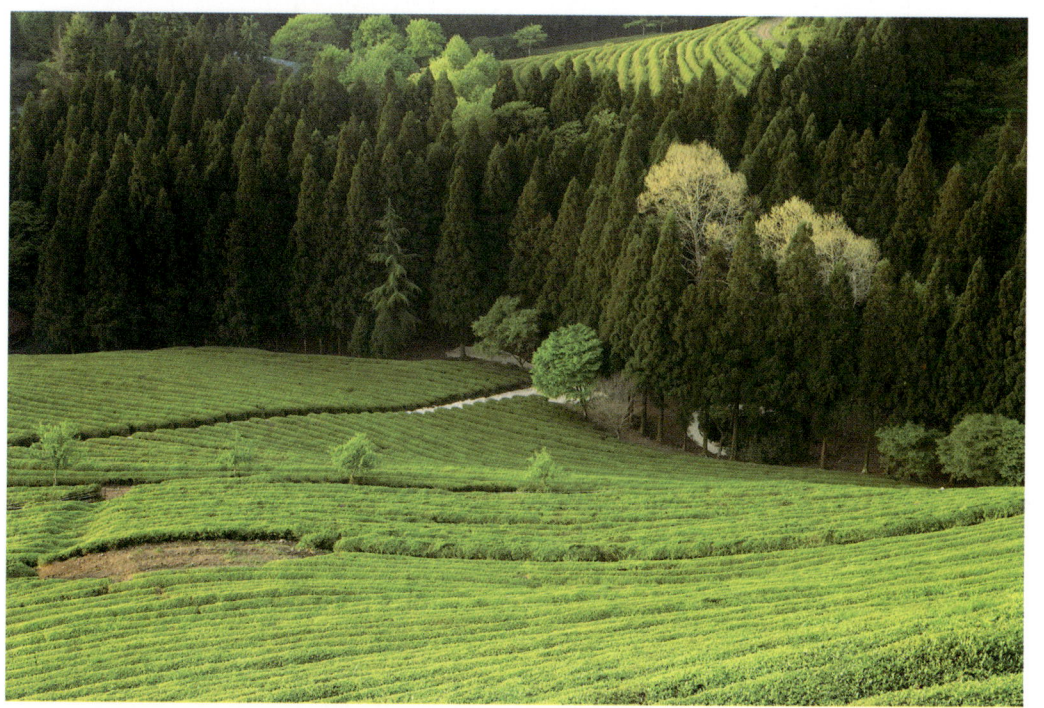

a relationship, one can expect the green lovers to be relaxed and innovative as well as adaptive. Their reputation and integrity is their defining trait and they are not the kind who will abandon a relationship or a task without seeing it to its end.

The one who loves green is a stable person with a warm, compassionate heart and such people make the best listeners in the whole world. They are inclined to be persistent and assertive as well as being frank and forthright about their views. Green lovers are hard working people who cope well with stress but can be stubborn about issues that mean a lot to them.

Yellow:

People whose favourite colour is yellow, the colour of the Sun, are quite like it too- with a sunny and cheerful disposition. They are blessed with an unusually witty sense of humour, are innovative intellectual with a fertile imagination and great business acumen. They have lofty ideas and make big claims but seldom see them through. They are spontaneous with comparatively short attention span. They crave mental stimulation and the one who can match their wits will be a suitable partner, who inturn, will be showered with unusual presents and equally quirky adventures.

A word of caution - these people are quite self obsessed. Though they are brimming with vitality and raw energy, romance and pleasing their partners does not top their list. They tend to be mental loners with a tendency of hastily changing a situation if it causes them grief or stress.

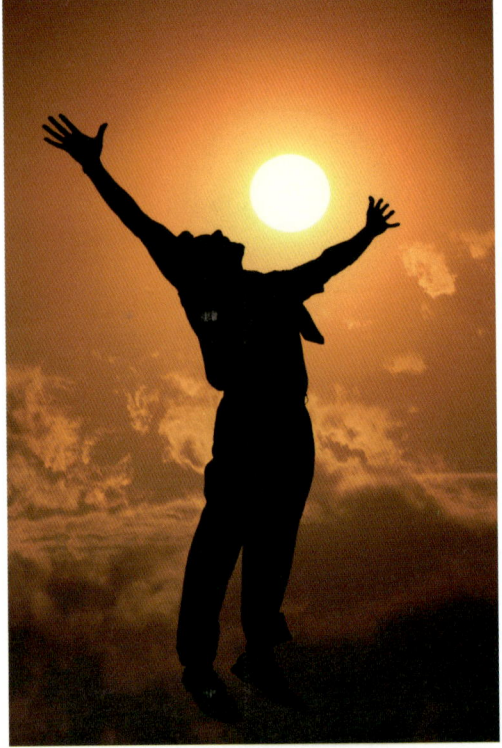

Orange:

This colour is the choice of a good natured and flamboyant person who loves an active social life. These people possess a generous heart and are very considerate. Being the colour of youth, people who like orange tend to remain young. Those around orange lovers can expect unconventional adventurous activities at all times.

Another trait of orange lovers, is that they can be a bit melodramatic and like to stand apart from the crowd. They are, at times, indecisive and inconsistent but they put in extra effort to be amicable and agreeable.

They are restless and always look out for someone who can match their zest for life. Once they forge a companionship with someone, they do not treat it lightly but remain loyal to the very end.

Such people are the connoisseurs of food and life and the best way to please them is to appease their gastronomic side or to involve them in fine works of art and poetry. Soft hearted and gentle, they take a while to open up but after that, it is a roller coaster ride all the way.

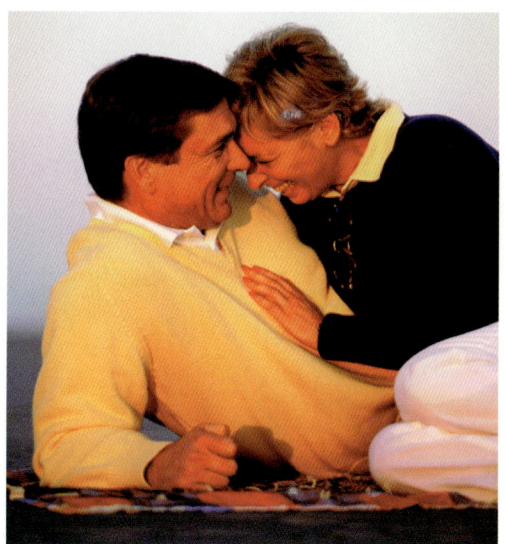

Red:

The colour of vitality and power, red is preferred by the outgoing extroverts or those who covet power and verve. They make the most of each moment and are largely optimistic.

They are also prone to complaining and what exasperates them the most is dreariness. Not given to serious introspection, people who like red occasionally have elevated peaks of energy and instant gratification is their mantra in life.

They possess remarkable will power and are inclined to experience every moment of life to the fullest. Given to mood swings, they have a particularly strong sex drive. They love to

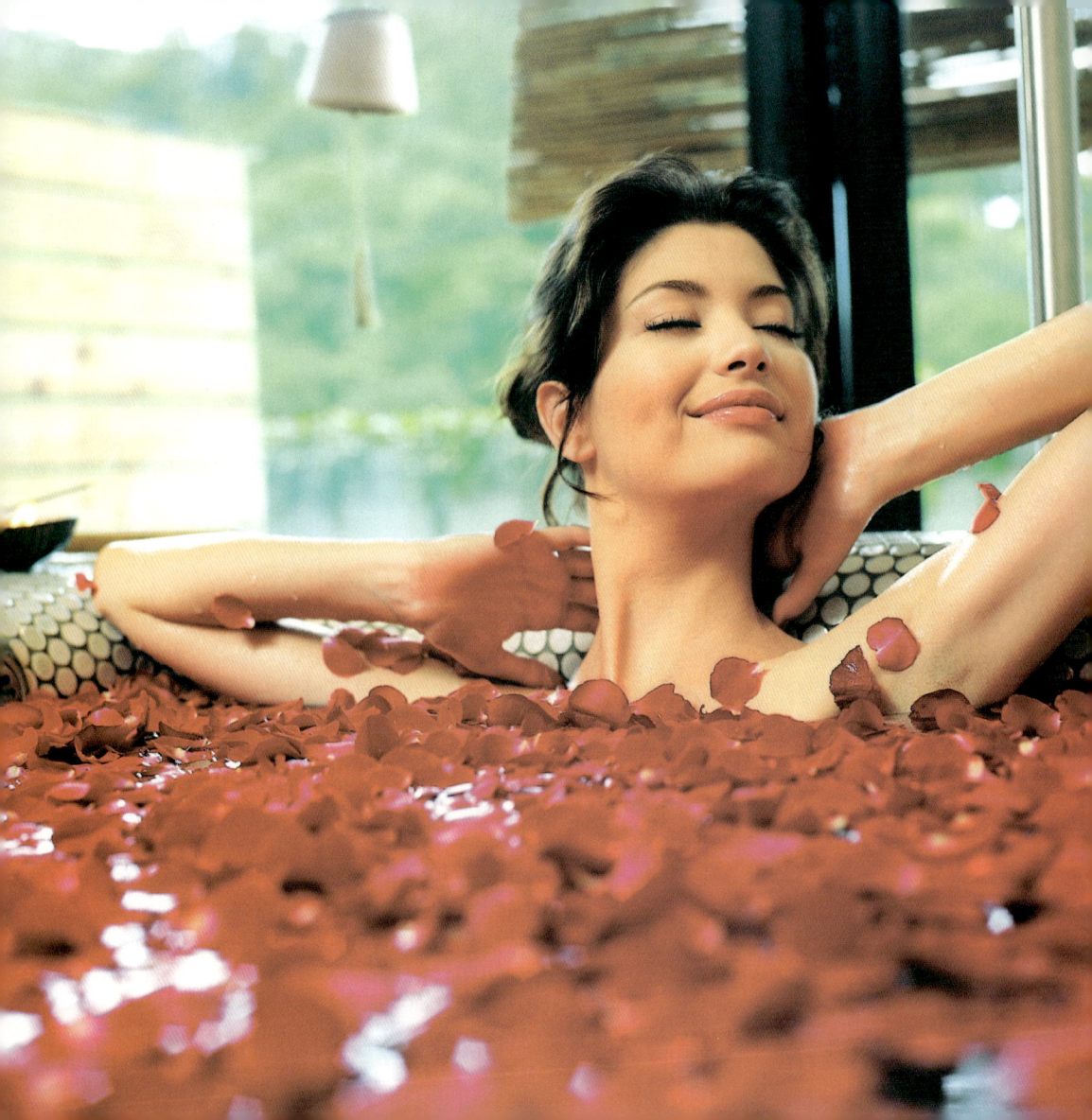

fantasize and so would probably jump into an extra marital affair but their strong sense of duty holds them back.

They have an uncomplicated nature and are the life of a party. If a relatively calm and sober person's favourite colour is red, it indicates that he/she aspires for the warmth and attention. Perhaps, beneath the quiet exterior lies a more passionate and fiery person.

Pink:

Those who have a strong bent towards pink are primarily gentle, charming, pleasant dreamers with a sweet disposition. They might at times be a bit indecisive about their actions.

These people seek romance in all aspects of their life. They desire a sense of security and protection. They love to be treated as special and fragile. Women who opt for pink, nurture an intense sense of maternity. They almost

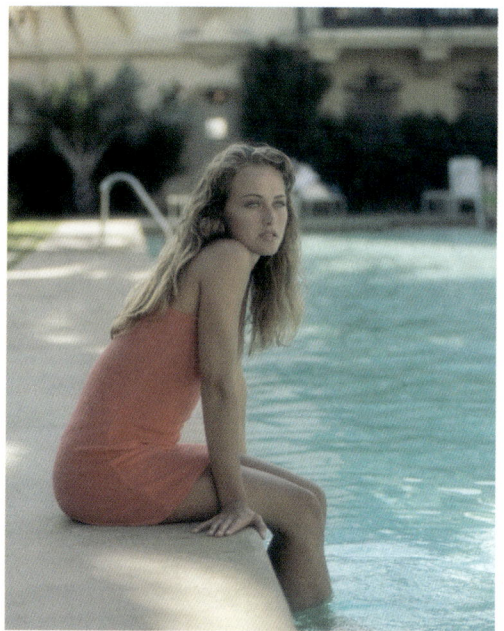
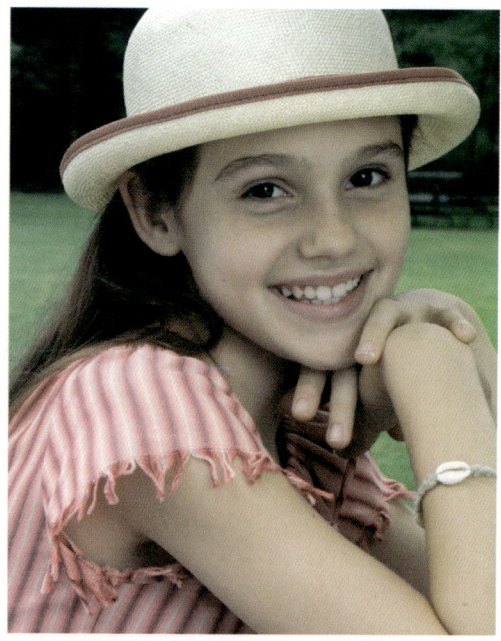

demand a sheltered life and, if given a chance, they would return to their days of innocence and childhood.

Brown:

The brown people are down-to-earth, trustworthy and intrinsically easy going. They would never pretend to be what they are not. Their priority is their home and family. Such persons are conscientious and aware of all their duties and responsibilities.

They are conservative, frugal with money and very astute business people. If in a relationship, one must expect them to be more thoughtful than lavish spenders.

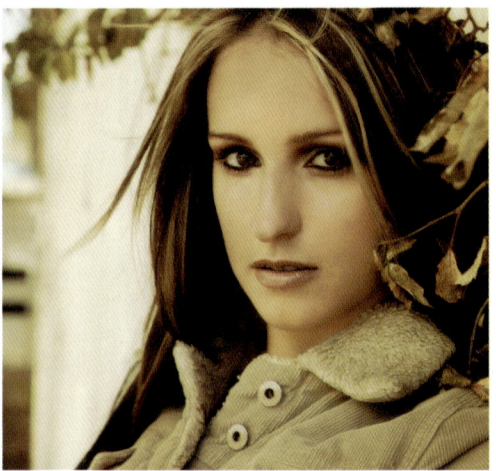

They possess a rare sense of patience and stamina due to which they always complete the tasks that are assigned or those they set themselves to. They love taking on responsibility but are also inflexible in their outlook.

These people are naturally inclined to love the outdoors and have a refined taste in art. They do not get swayed by new trends and prefer to remain with their sense of the familiar. They can therefore conveniently be labelled as 'old school'.

Grey:

People who prefer grey to other colours strive for peace and quietude. They are exceptionally hard working who often go without being rewarded. They are reserved, who refrain from active participation in social activities. They would rather sit back and watch the turn of events passively. The fondness of grey in a person reveals that he/she chooses to withdraw from social activities and never interfere with other peoples' lives.

Being relaxed and mild, they can make good friends with everyone if they wish to. They have a keen eye for aesthetics and excel in arts. Although they appear to be in control of situations, they are constantly looking in words and appraising the situations around them.

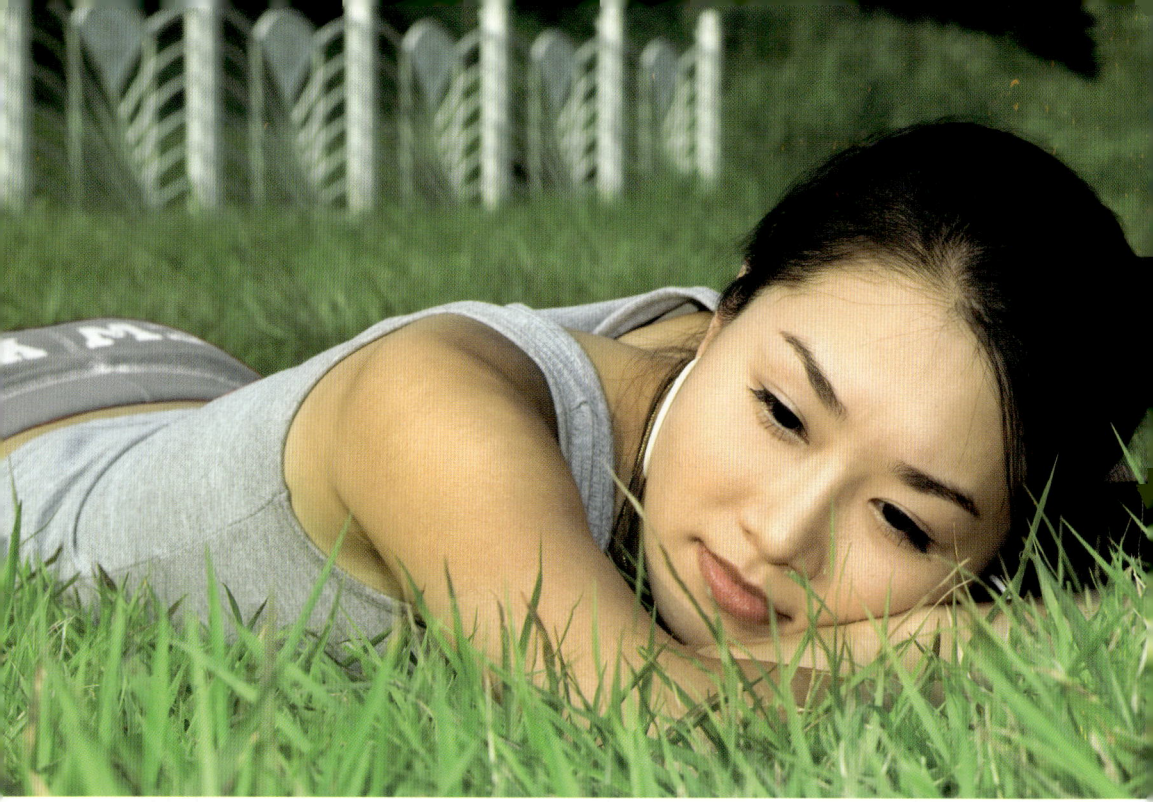

Black:

Black, quite like white is a combination of all the seven colours of the spectrum, but while white represents peace and serenity, black conveys that those who prefer this colour the most are experienced, poised and stately above all. The black lovers demand attention and at the same time come across as mysterious who mostly leave people intrigued and wanting to know more about them.

The black folk are unconventional, they have an inquisitive mind and are natural born leaders. They dislike being accountable to anyone and love leading an adventurous life. People who like black want others around

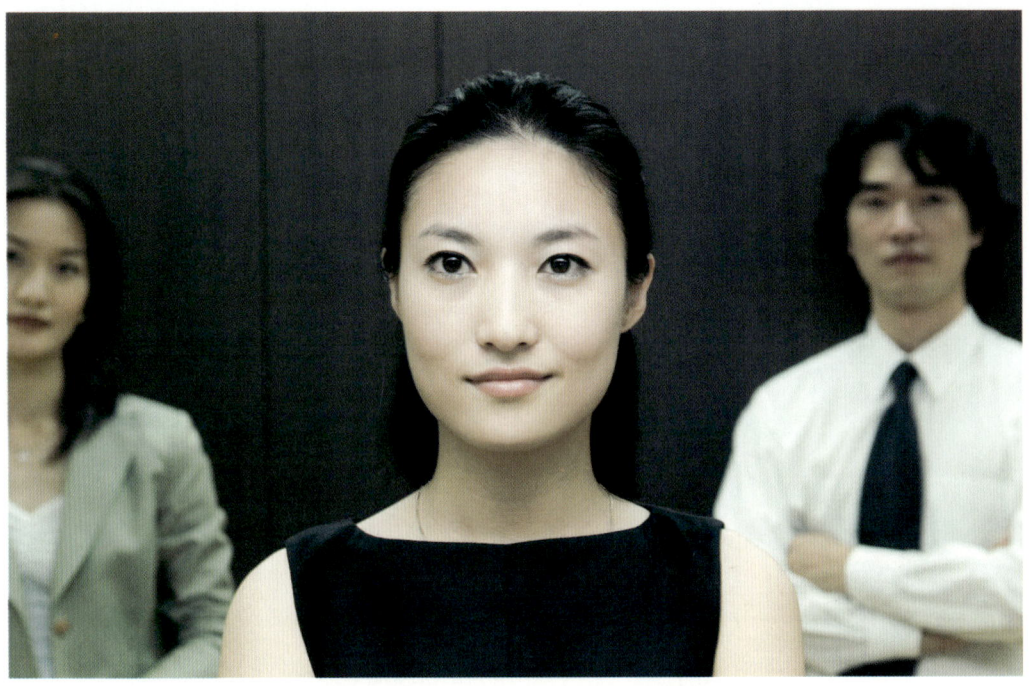

them to be forthright since they themselves are very candid. To have him/her love one endlessly, all one needs to do is be sincere and everything else simply falls into place for them These people may be suppressing their desires and inner longings and harbour magnificent visions of a fulfilling life. Such people abhor disagreements but at the same time do not get thrown off balance easily.

Chapter 5
COLOUR COMPATIBILITY

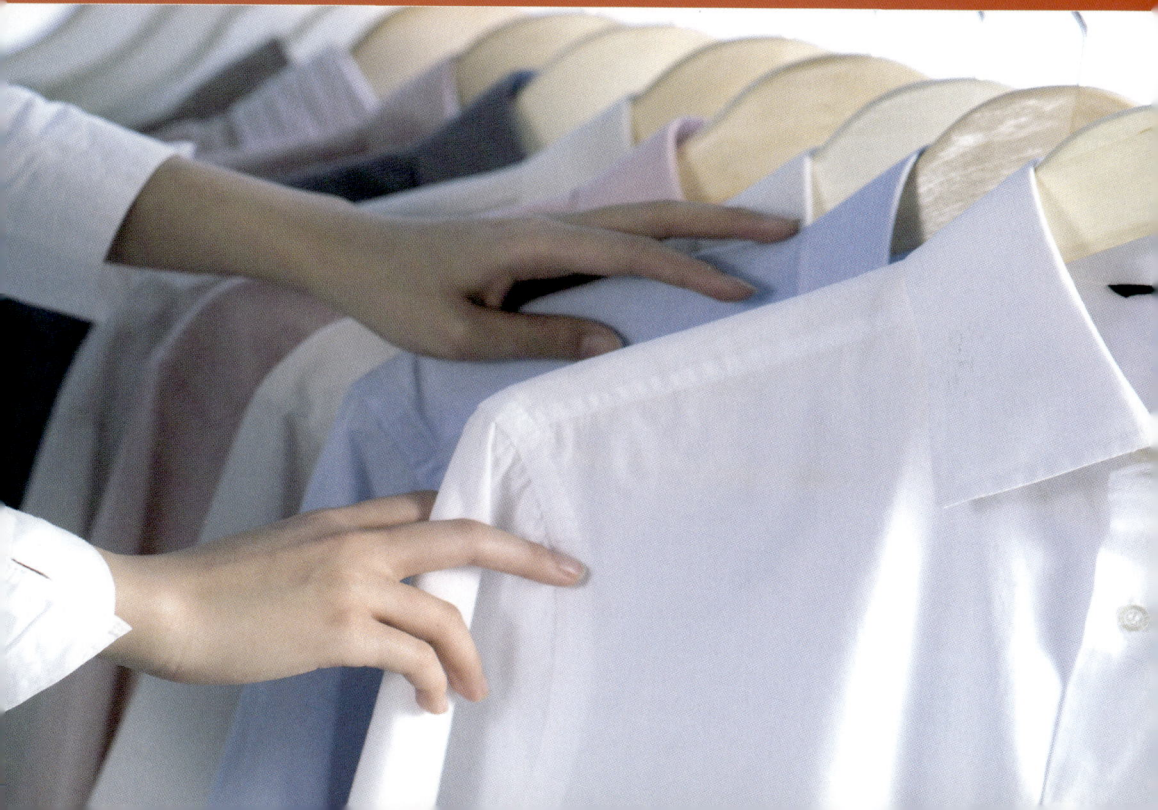

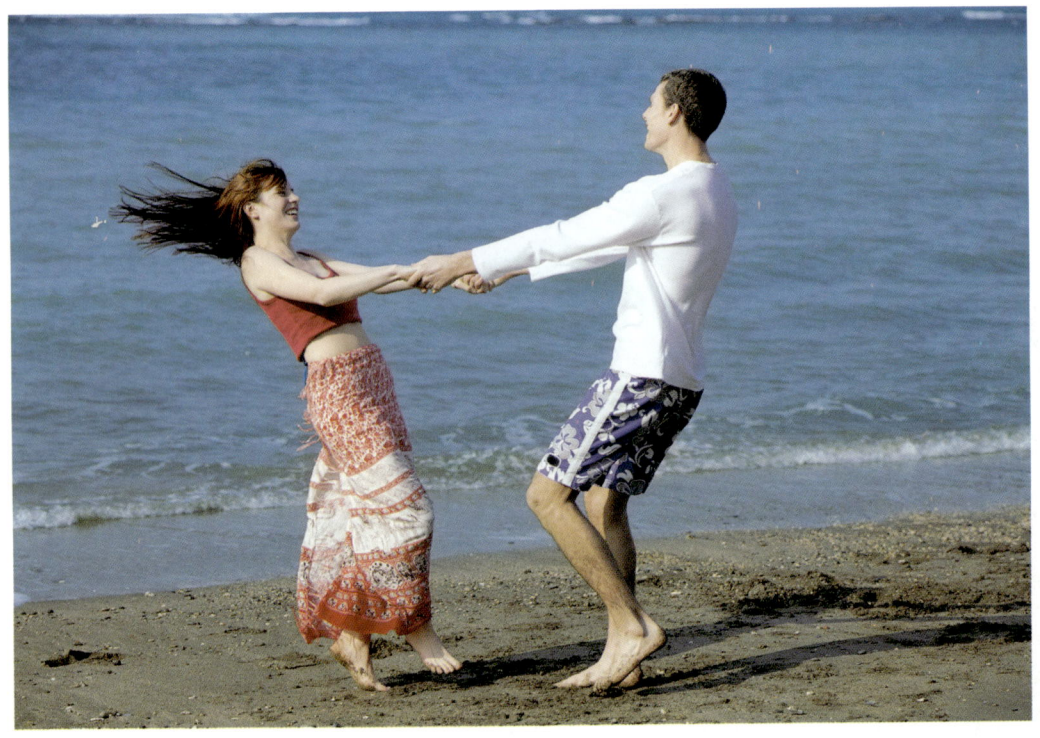

Red and White:

As a couple, the red person may outrun the white partner in the quest for adventure and the hunger for experimentation in life while the latter may want to stop a while to take in the natural beauty around him/her. As much as the red person may want unbounded love making in many positions, the white person is mostly blissfully wedded to the missionary position. While the red person might just add a hint of dynamism that is lacking in a white person's otherwise almost perfect life, the white partner could ground the red half into a state of harmony and balance.

Colour Compatibility

Red and Violet:

A violet person has a sharp wit that tends to make the red sit up and notice. The red ones like to be with people who can always keep them on their toes and fuel their desire for exploration.

As a couple, they are fine-tuned owing to the fact that the purple folk love anything that is superlative and inimitable and the red people seem to echo the same thought. In bed to, they score high points because of their inherent flair and ability to experiment and discover each other over and over again. Such a relationship can bring great joy to the lovers provided they do not get into too many heated arguments because both have strong opinions and can be stubborn about their view points.

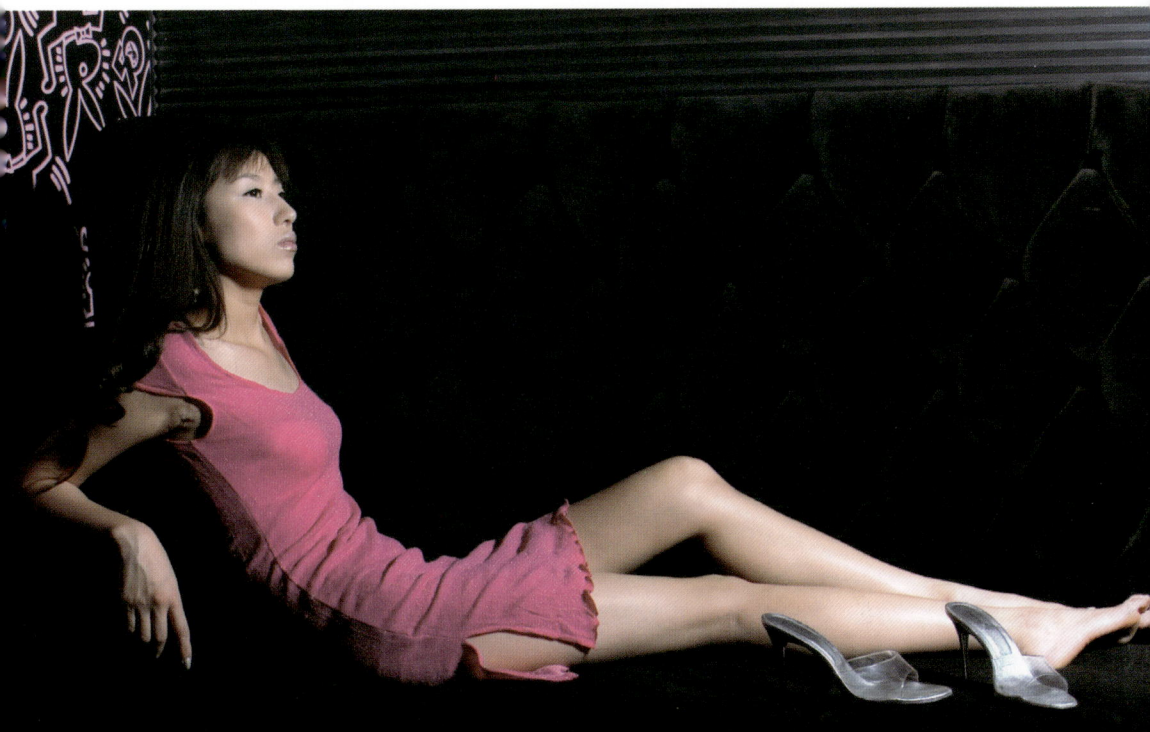

Red and Blue:

This combination scores the most over anything in terms of physical love. Both the red and blue persons demonstrate their love physically, be it hugging their partner or making sensual love for long unending hours.

The blue person is a dreamer. Many of their dreams do not get to see the light of the day which might irk the go-getter red who is in constant quest for power, fame and prestige. The blue person is also given to excesses, which might raise the red partner's temper which is mercurial but quells just as easily. A dynamic relationship at the end of the day which is inspiring as well as exciting.

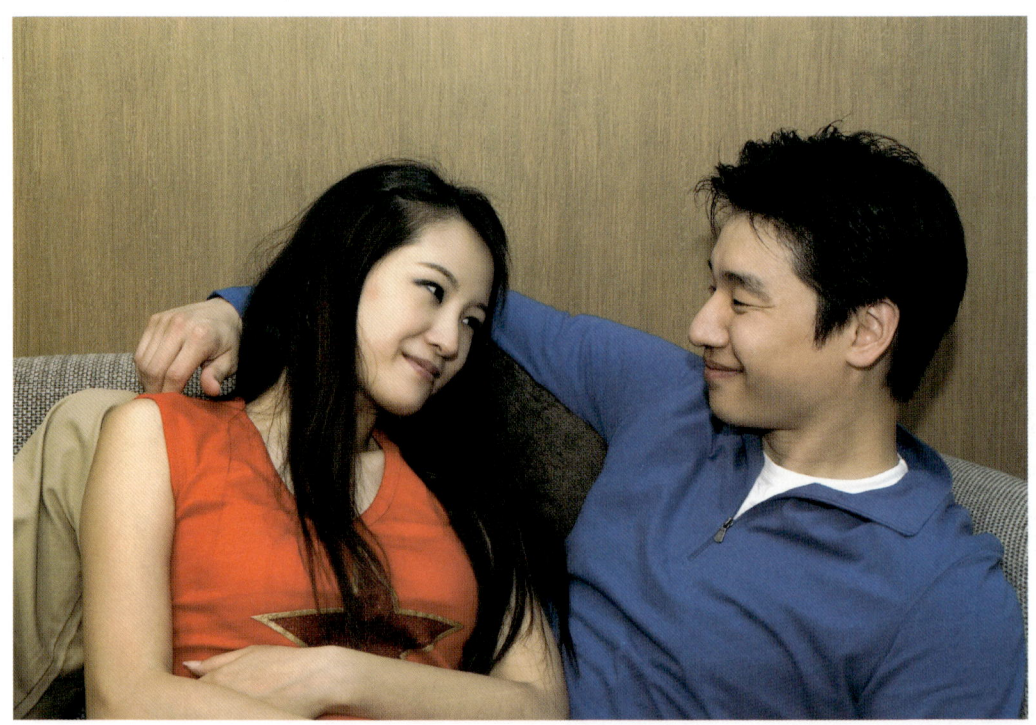

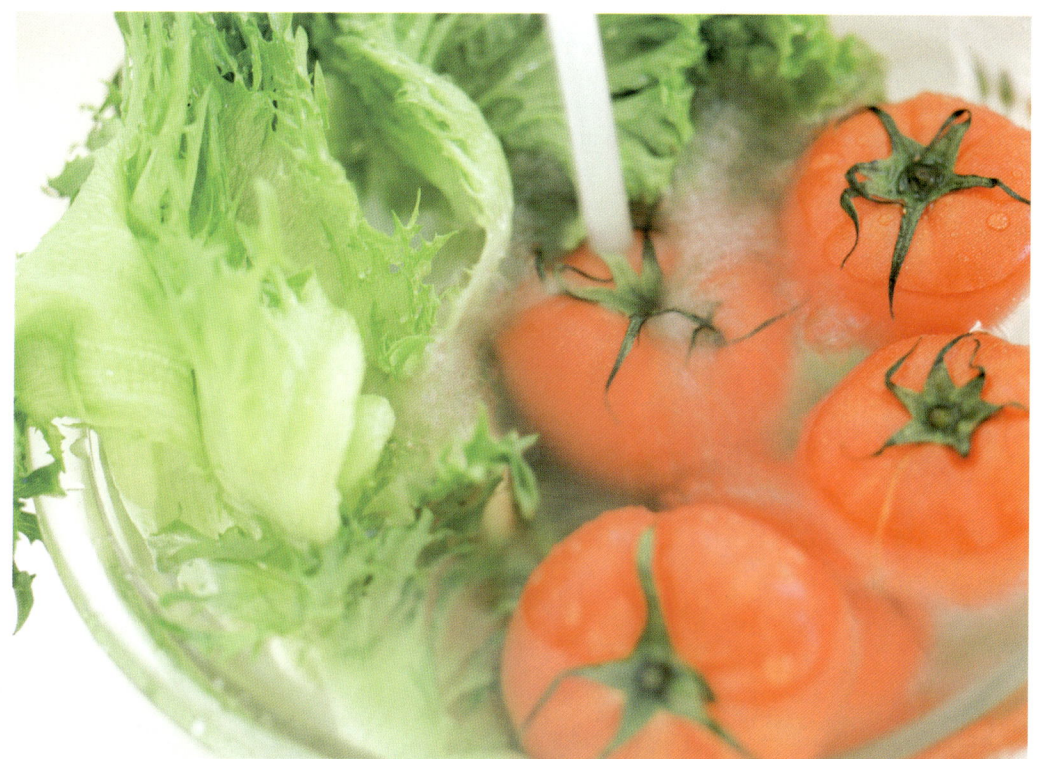

Red and Green:

The red people are creative in all fields. They rush to set tasks for themselves and then are in a frantic hurry to accomplish them. The green people, on the other hand are basically contended beings who like a relaxed pace of life which enables them to enjoy the beauty of life. The quality to give in these people from emotions to love making can actually enhance the charitable side of the red person and adds to the stability in their relationship.

Red and Yellow:

Innovation and intellect are the key traits of a yellow person. He is always looking out for some intelligent means of recreation and in that sense, they find their best buddy in a red person who is also witty and dynamic. The flip side is that both the red and yellow folk are generally quite self centred which might result in ego clashes and lack of togetherness. Therefore, the relationship between red and yellow might need a bit of effort to make it work but once started, it can be a sizzling hot relationship.

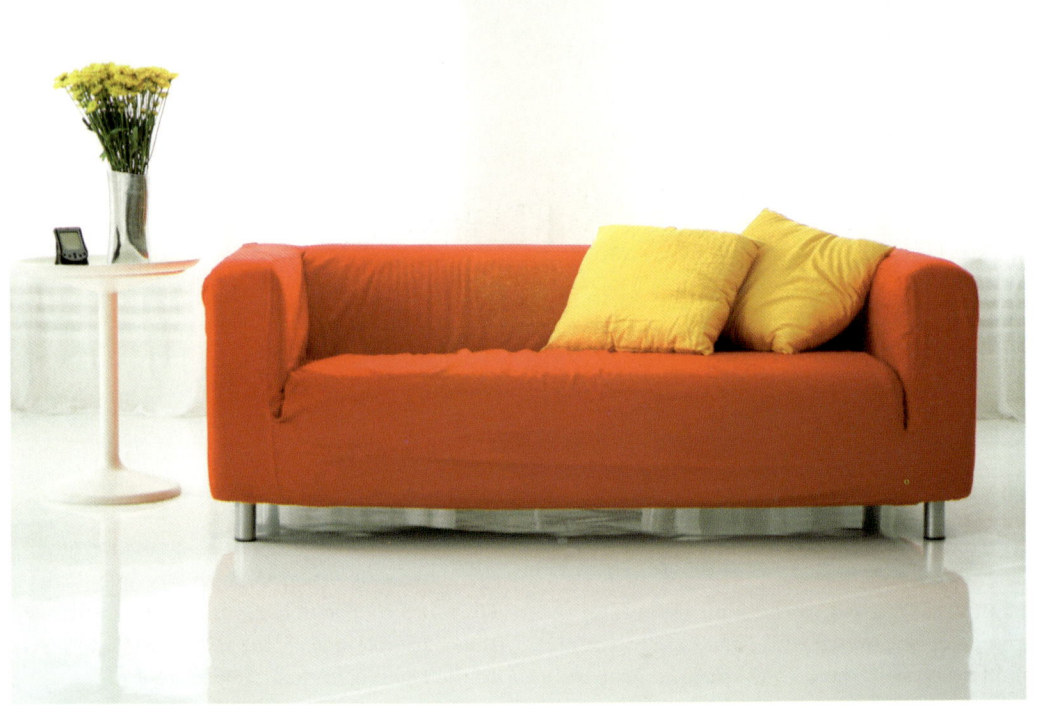

Red and Orange:

The orange person is cheerful, sunny, adventurous with a hint of cinematic melodrama. This is exactly what attracts the vivacious red people to the orange folk. The red person's undoing is that when monotony sets into a relationship, it makes him/her want to search elsewhere simply because a drab environment is intolerable to him/her. With an orange person's crazy antics, there is least likelihood of this happening. It works just as well for the orange folk who too cannot bear the dullness of a monotonous relationship. Both red and orange people love the luxuries of life. When together, they look in the same direction. Working out a relationship is no problem since they both have so much in common that things rarely ever go wrong.

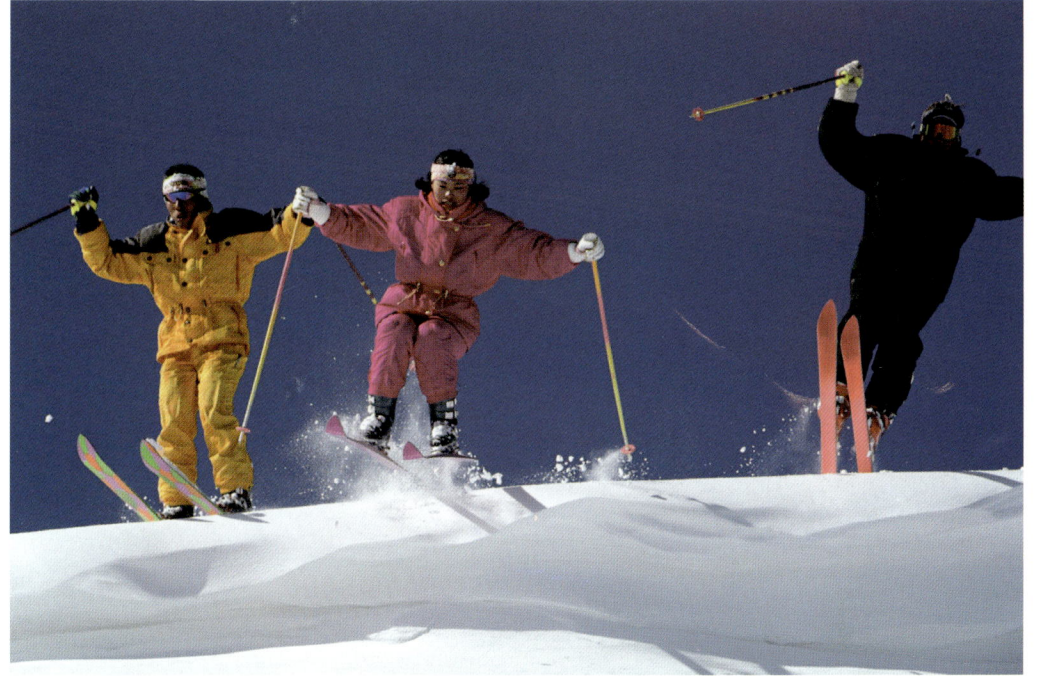

Red and Pink:

The red folk are always in a frantic rush wanting to try out life in all its facets while the pink ones are leisurely. Though pink is a derivative of red, the only thing that red and pink people have in common is that they both appreciate and indulge in a healthy and robust romantic life. However, that is where the similarities end. While the red folk want more pizzazz and action, the pink people are content with a little in life that is abounding in romance.

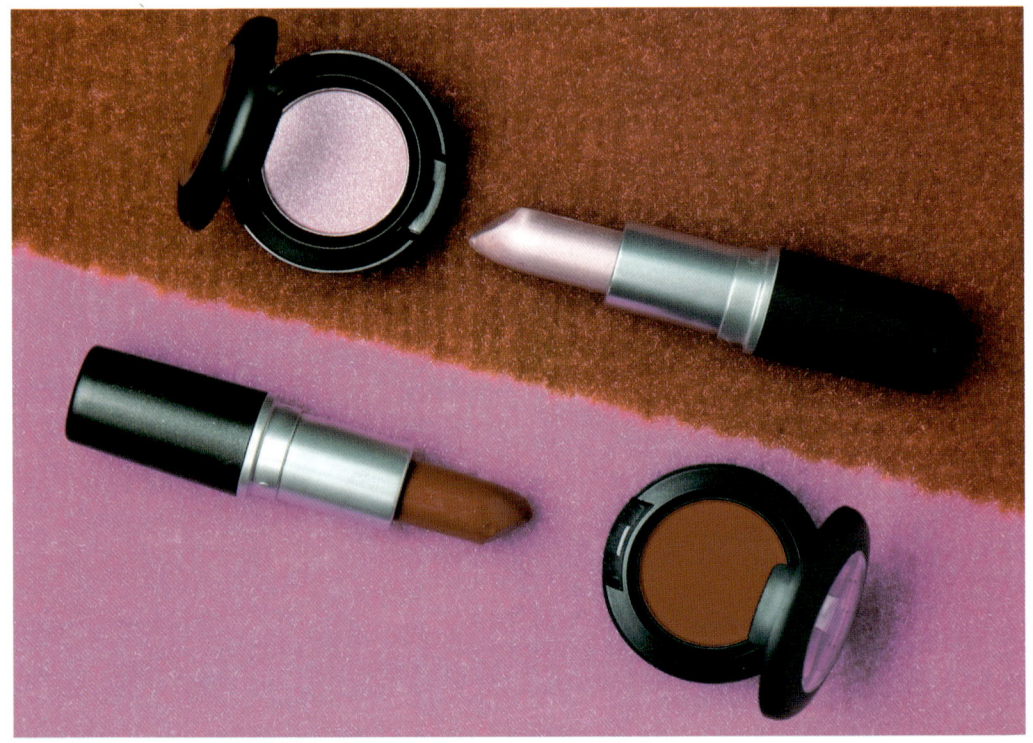

Colour Compatibility

Red and Brown:

Red and brown are beautiful colours when juxtaposed with each other but when red and brown people meet, a great deal of friction is expected. The brown people are a grounded type, level-headed and practical while the red ones are enthusiastic and impulsive. They are bound to disapprove of each other in most situations.

This romance will work only in one case: if the red person has 'been there, done that' and finally wishes to settle down. In such a situation, a brown person can lend a supportive and sturdy companionship and conversely, if the brown person wishes to transform his/her conventional lifestyle, then the red person is the perfect choice.

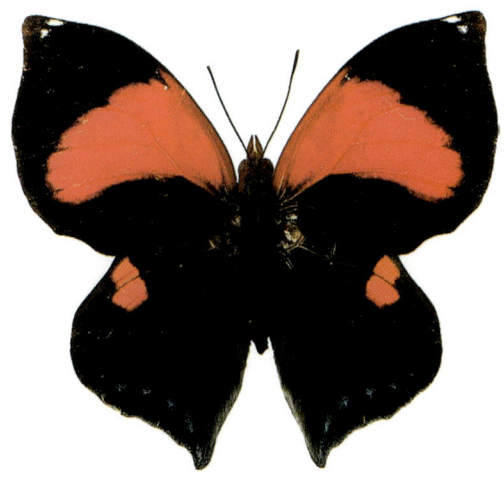

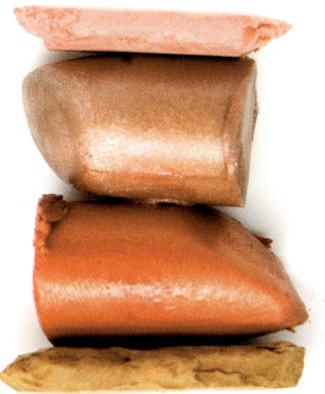

Red and black:

Red and black, a conventionally classic colour combination translates into an equally classic relationship. Both are attention- loving: they love the spotlight to be on them and they both have an insatiable thirst for matchless things, be it emotions or the experience of living. They both have a magnificent vision of being leaders and each fuels the other's lust for life.

In every way, a dynamic relationship, there will never be a dull moment in their lives and the only thing to watch out for is the fact that they might get involved in some serious disagreements with each other.

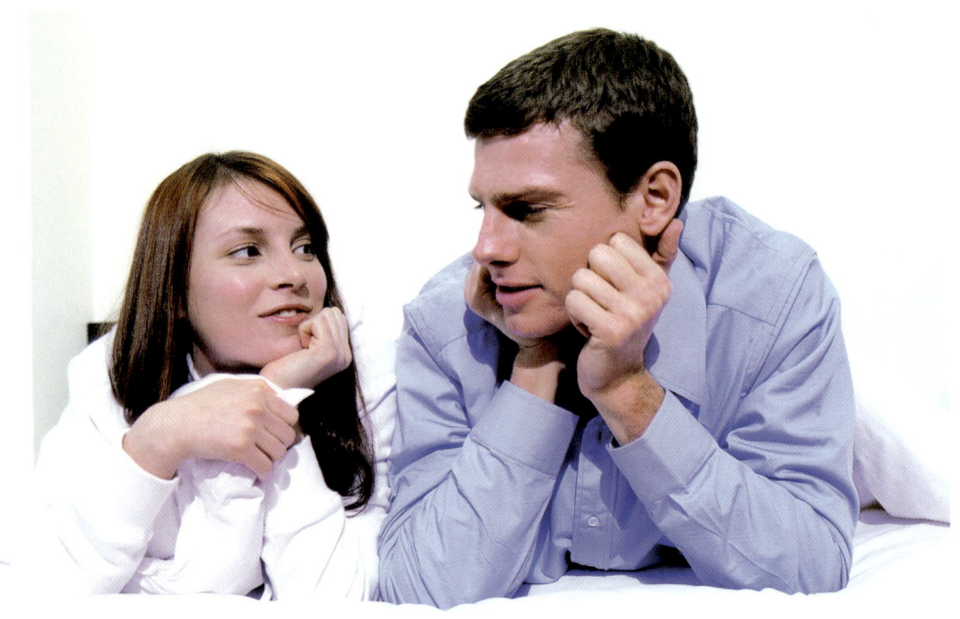

White and Purple:

The white and purple is an ideal combination. Both are kind, thoughtful and intelligent. Moreover, these are the very qualities that both look for in their mate. They are both affectionate, quixotic and can spend hours listening to old melodious tunes on a gramophone if they can lay their hands on one. Chances are that they will probably meet at an antique shop or an old forgotten bookstore.

A word of caution : when the purple person is irked, he/she can be quite verbose, which in turn will disturb the white partner who believes in sorting out a situation amicably.

White and Blue:

This is a combination that can throw the white personality into a tizzy; the blue person is generally compassionate and tender but sometimes tends to drift away into a world of his/her own, leaving the simple and the undemanding white person feeling neglected. Other than that, they share their love for the uncomplicated and languid life in which they can read out poetry to each other and feel that their world is complete. The good thing about this particular combination is that, like wine, they both get better with age. If together for a long time, they begin to resemble each other.

White and Green:

White and green are colours found in abundance in nature and they complement each other perfectly. This equation spills over in the life of the white and green couple as well. Both want to give so much of themselves to please their partner that, at times they wish for a partner who would enjoy receiving all the favours. Both the white and green persons are easygoing, tolerant, kind and never forget a good turn. They love to mingle with people and share all that they have and so, make excellent hosts. Both desire a secure family life, which they find in each other's companionship.

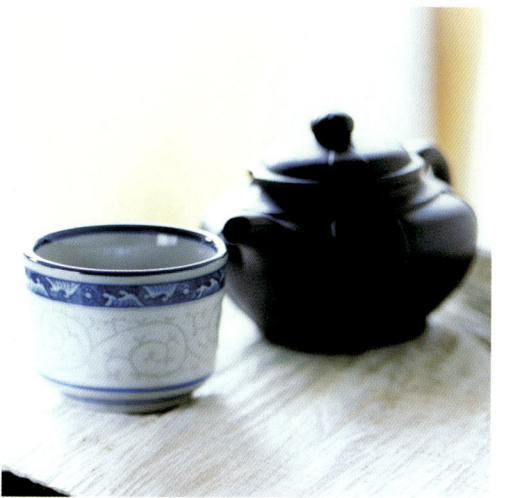

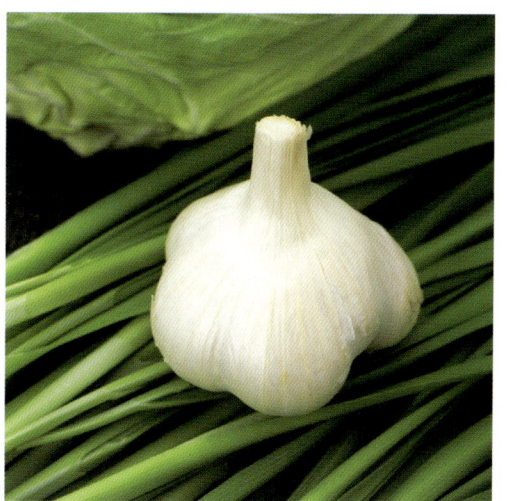

White and Yellow:

This is a somewhat crazy combination because the white personality is a sombre one, looking for little and finding great satisfaction in what he/she has. The yellow ones, on the other hand, are always looking for something different. Things that are out of the ordinary. The white folk, conversely, are happy being conformists and conventional. The yellow people may annoy the white people who detest unpredictability.

A difficult but not impossible partnership, that can work if the white person is willing to experience adventure with the same spirit and the yellow person is ready to rein his/her frenzied quest for the outlandish.

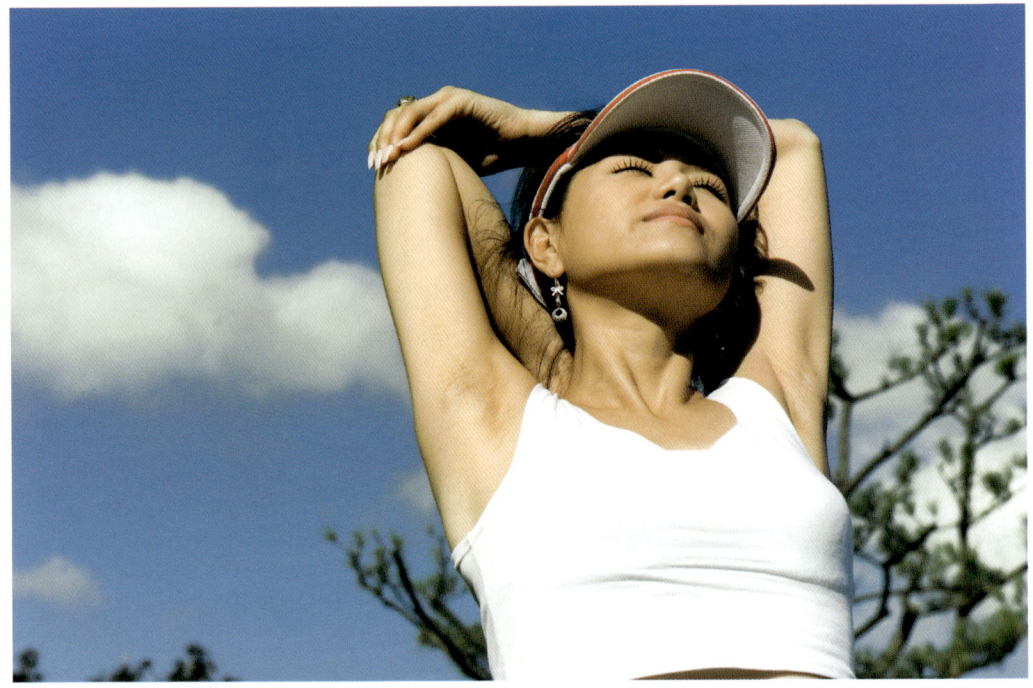

Colour Compatibility

White and Orange:

Always wanting to be admired, an orange person is flamboyant which makes him/her the life of a party and the funny person in the office, due to a hint of eccentricity in his/her nature. These very traits, however, upset the conservative white person who delves in the depth of silence and stillness. He/she never craves attention. Only if the white person is looking out for a whiff of freshness, he/she might welcome the orange person. Moreover, the orange person who is looking for stability and tranquillity, found in plenitude in a white person, will be content in this relationship.

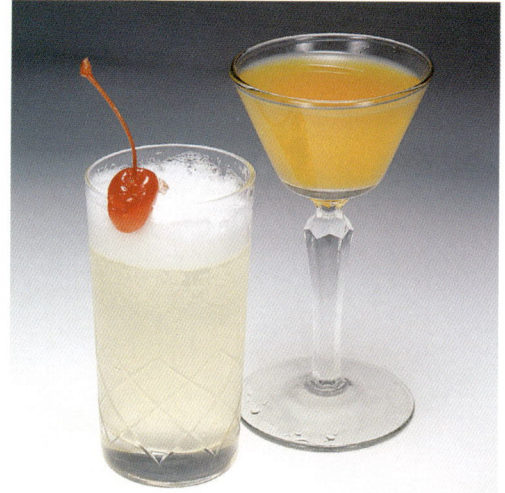

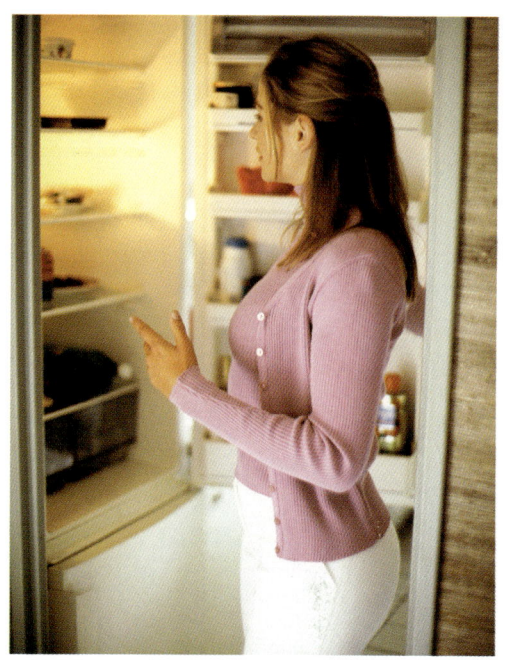

White and Pink:

The pink personality is timid and reticent who doesn't like to mingle with the people much, is happy reading Victorian literature and always looking out for a perfect love story in books and in his/her own life. The white personality, to him/her comes as the hero or heroine that the pink person seeks. The orderly white person is an epitome of tranquillity which the pink person greatly appreciates. Together, the two can find themselves a love nest anywhere and spend a great deal of time discussing philosophy or narrating love stories to each other.

White and Brown:

The white and brown couple is well-suited to each other. The brown person is family-oriented who looks for a stable relationship at the very onset. The white person's sense of commitment puts the brown partner, almost immediately, at ease. A white person, on the other hand, is constantly searching for someone who can add more substance to his/her life. The brown person does just that without any flippancy. They are both fond of the finer things of life. In each other they, not only find great companionship but also the best of friendship.

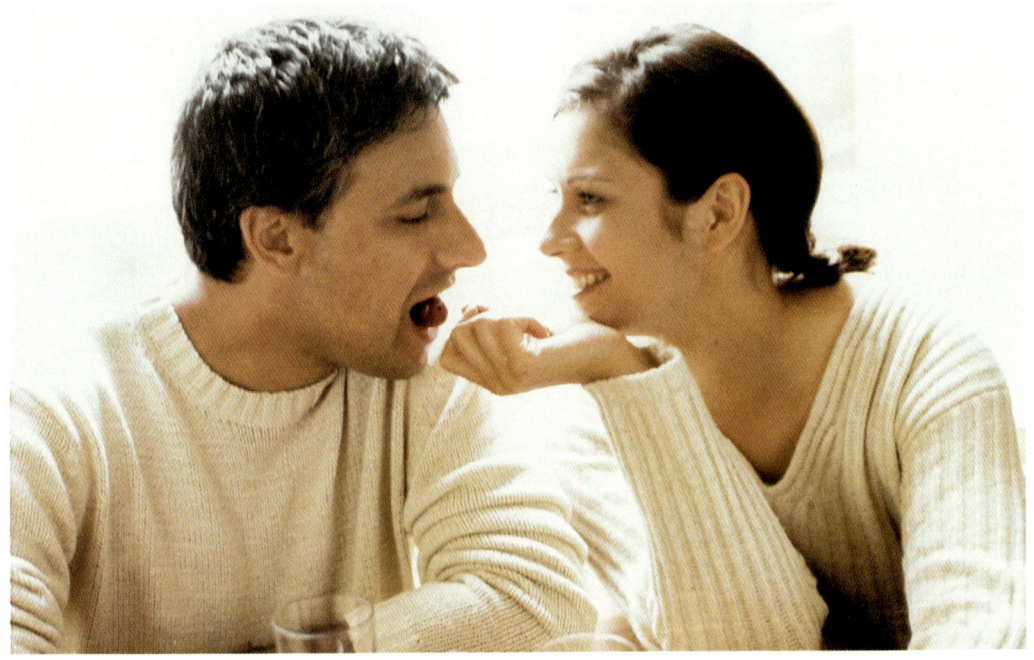

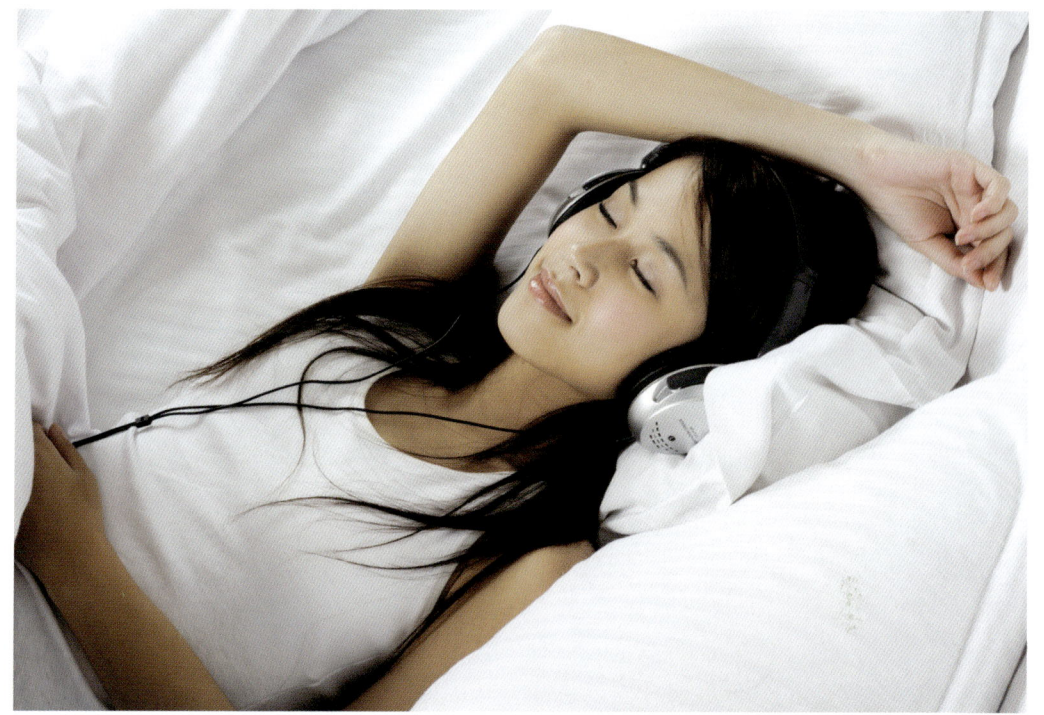

White and Black:

A classic combination from the perspective of design but when a black and white person meet, they are poles apart. While the white personality likes silence and serenity, the black personality seeks the spotlight and has an insatiable desire to establish his/her credibility as a leader. The white people are unhurried and lyrical while the black ones are articulate and lucid in both their thinking and expression. The two have little in common. The only commonality is that both tend to suppress their real feelings about life which they can best discuss with each other.

Purple and Blue:

The purple personality is bewildered by the blue person's penchant for animated conversation and his/her ability to stand and smell the roses. All this fascinates the purple person who finds anything out of the ordinary, a source of great wonder. The blue person, on the contrary, realises his/her dream of stability in a purple person whose commitment is final and binding. This relationship has the makings of an epic romance, not so much in terms of passion but due to the power game that these two indulge in. Many unexpected twists and turns are the hallmarks of this relationship. The only hitch is that, after a point, the relationship can reach a deadend as both tend to lose direction after a while.

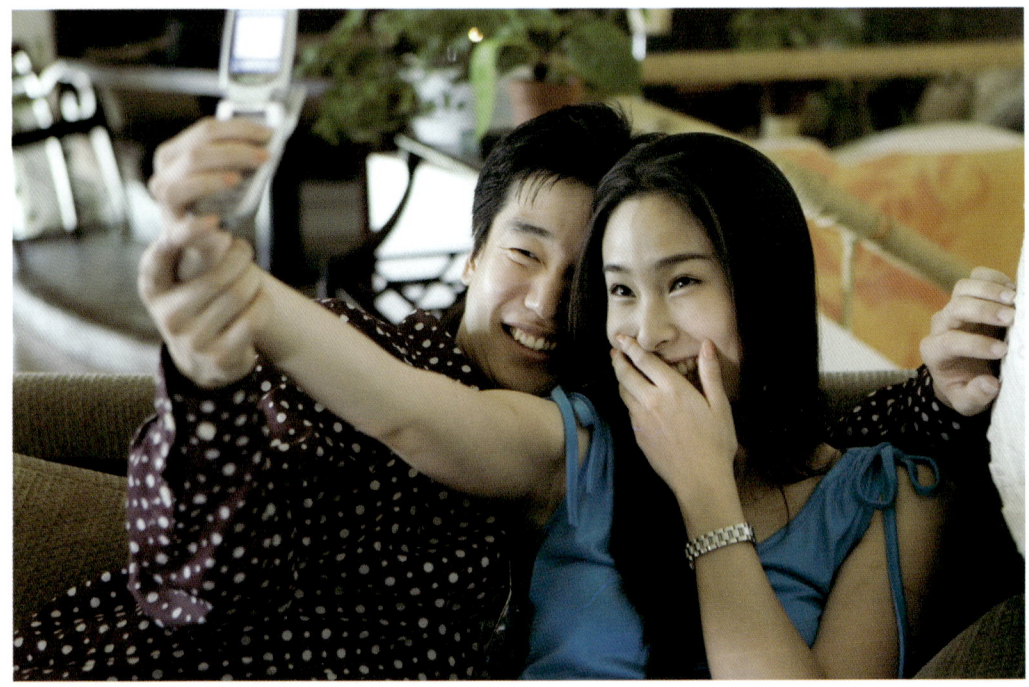

Colour Compatibility

Purple and Green:

The green person is a conformist who loves to be a melting pot of all things considered politically- correct and morally-upright. The purple person, on the other hand, is just the opposite. An individualist, his/her mantra is to stand apart from the crowd. This couple in all likelihood, would start with a heady brew of troubles. The reason why a purple person would seek a green personality is because of his/her desire for a secure home and hearth. The green persons would be addicted to the purple folk due to their intrigue quotient which never ceases to fascinate the green ones. However, this relationship would require sincere efforts to make it work.

Purple and Yellow:

The effervescent yellow personality is dreamy and bubbling with life while the purple person observes and appreciates the minutest qualities of things, which most people fail to notice. This is exactly what brings the two together: the purple person loves the gay abandon of the yellow person and conversely, the yellow personality is inspired by the graces and compassion of the purple. The purple person has the ability to make the yellow person remain on the 'terra firma' while the yellow person fuels the ambitions and aspirations of the purple person.

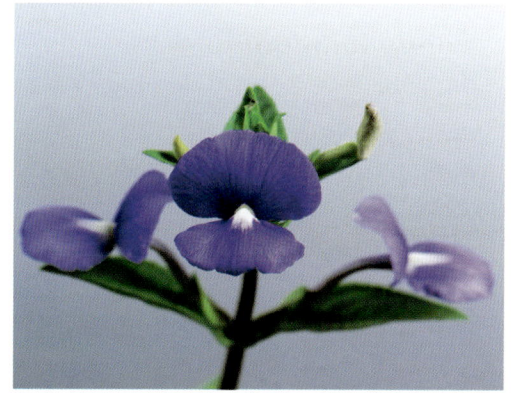

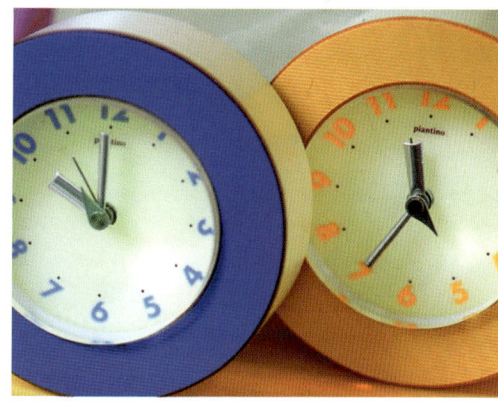

Purple and Orange:

The purple and orange persons make a very compatible match in all respects. Both the personalities seek like-minded people and they find just that in each other. The purple person finds the orange personality emotionally, mentally and physically stimulating. The purple partner is in her/his element in the inspiring company of the orange folk who. inturn, fuel the fantasies of their partner. This is a highly active and lively combination which has all the ingredients of making a quintessential tale of romance that culminates in a stable and satisfying marriage.

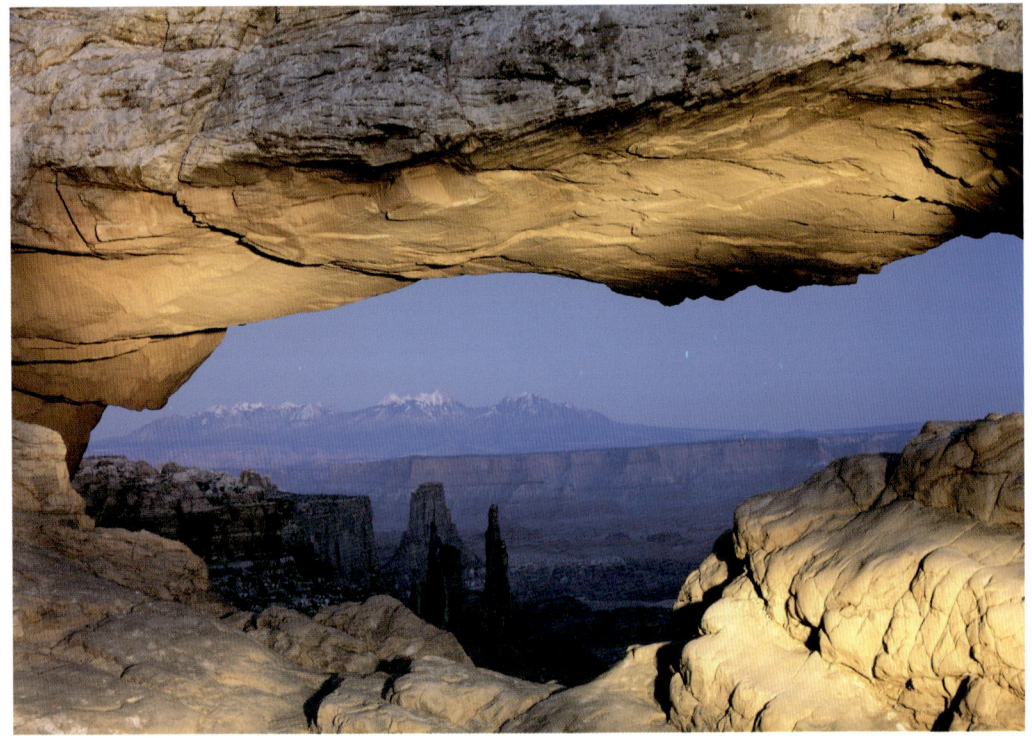

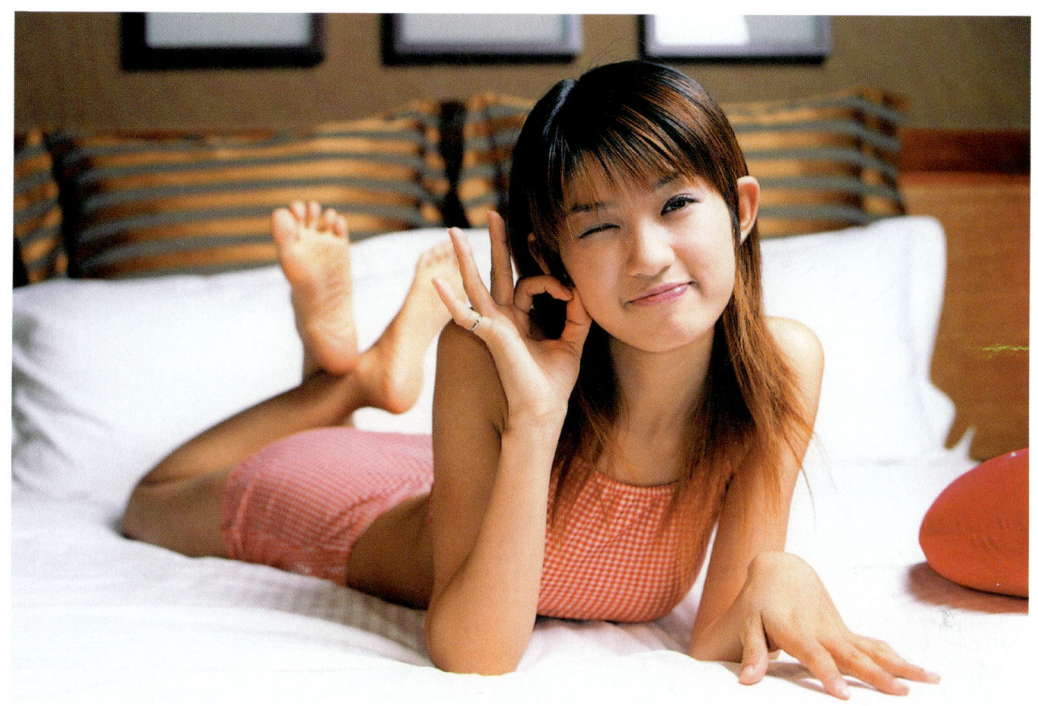

Purple and Pink:

Purple and pink is a pretty combination, a favourite with the young girls. A relationship between these two personality types is just as pretty. The pink personality is a fragile one, looking for protection in a relationship and when the purple person senses this need, he/she becomes very protective. The pink person is the happiest when sheltered emotionally and physically. The purple person can spend his/her entire life ensuring that everything is just perfect for the pink partner. All the giving and receiving in this relationship is based on the one thing that they both have in abundance: romance and ample time for it.

Purple and Brown:

This combination works best for a business proposition. The purple person spends lavishly and the brown folk is just as frugal with money and hence, the balance. However, in an emotional relationship, there can be plenty of obstacles to be overcome. Both the brown and purple personalities love the home and the hearth but the purple person's constant quest for the unusual can sometimes exasperate the brown personality, who would prefer to spend time gardening than searching for old and dusty things in an antique shop. The brown person's old and conventional approach to almost all things could get the couple into ideological differences. A match that would rather be termed a mismatch would have many problems but there would also be some special moments.

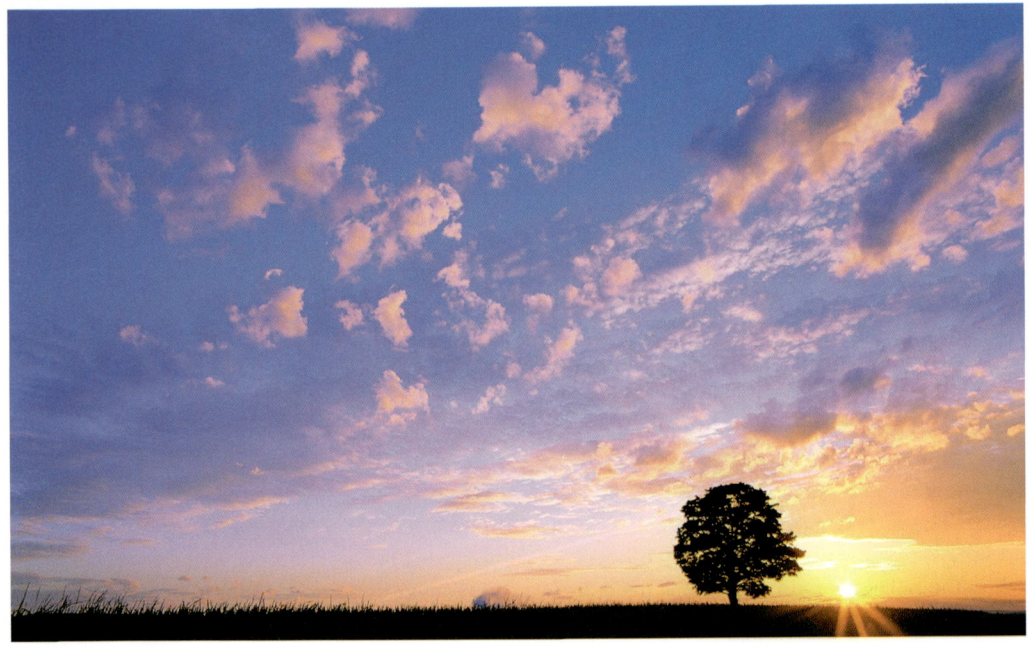

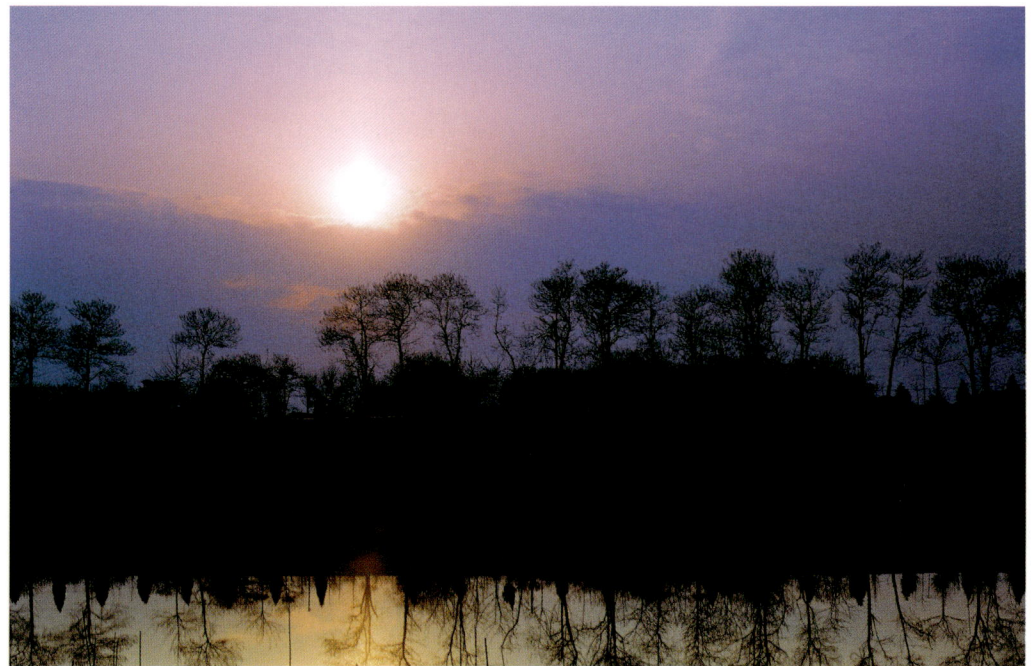

Purple and Black:

A very surreal combination, the black and purple are each others best friends and can make very loyal lovers. Both are highly individualistic people who debate often on issues and yet revel in disagreeing. A relationship between the purple and the black people will be based on lots of deliberations and pondering over metaphysical and philosophical issues and yet they can sit over coffee with such a smug feeling of oneness as if they had never disagreed. The black person does not like accountability and the purple person does not ask for it. The black person completely intrigues the purple person with his/her sense of mystery and magic and that ensures that the relationship is a long lasting one.

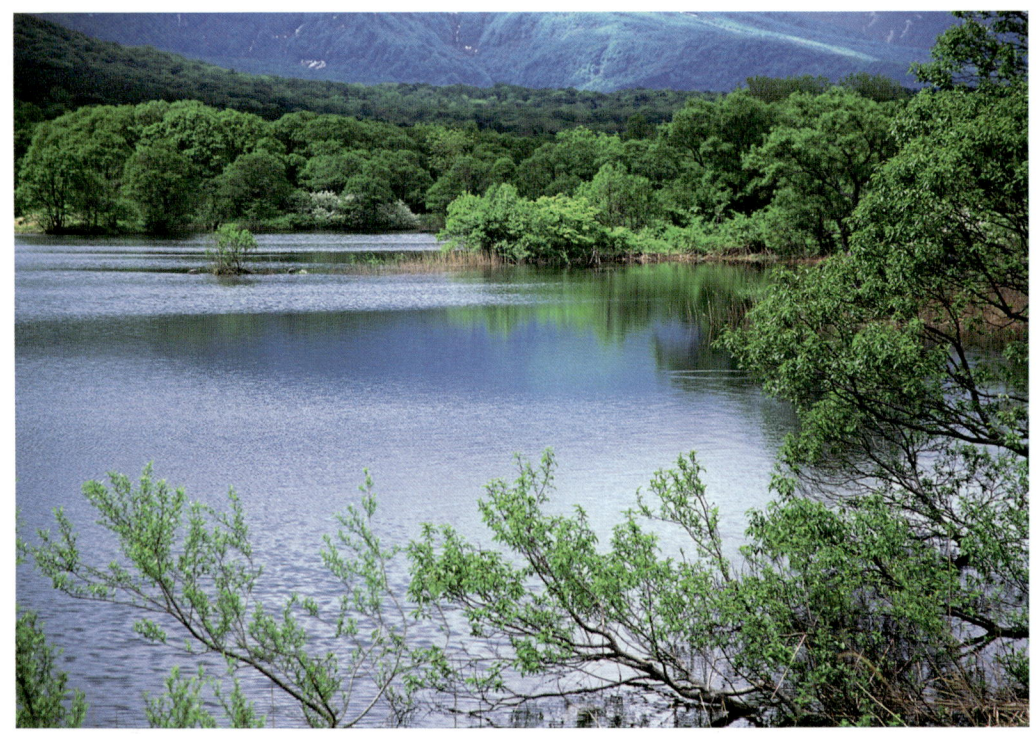

Blue and Green:

Quite like the green grass merging with the blue skies at the horizon, the green and blue personalities have a lot in common. Both are meditative and sombre with the traits of a connoisseur thrown in good measure. Chances are that this couple will be seen often at a restaurant, enjoying a quiet evening with some vintage wine, oblivious to the world. The blue and green personalities are subtly drawn to the unknown and the mysterious, both reaching out to be one with the energies of the cosmos. Essentially a satisfying and balanced relationship that will remain snug and cosy forever.

Colour Compatibility

Blue and Yellow:

The blue and yellow persons are constantly at loggerheads. The blue person is tranquil and peace loving while the sunny yellow person is always raring to go. The yellow person can force the blue one to travel and explore which may not be desirable to the yellow person.

The blue person, on the other hand, would try and make the yellow person temperate which he/she may resent. The blue person would demand accountability which the yellow would not tolerate. However, the couple may learn a lot from each other's diverse personalities but the conflict can take its toll on the relationship.

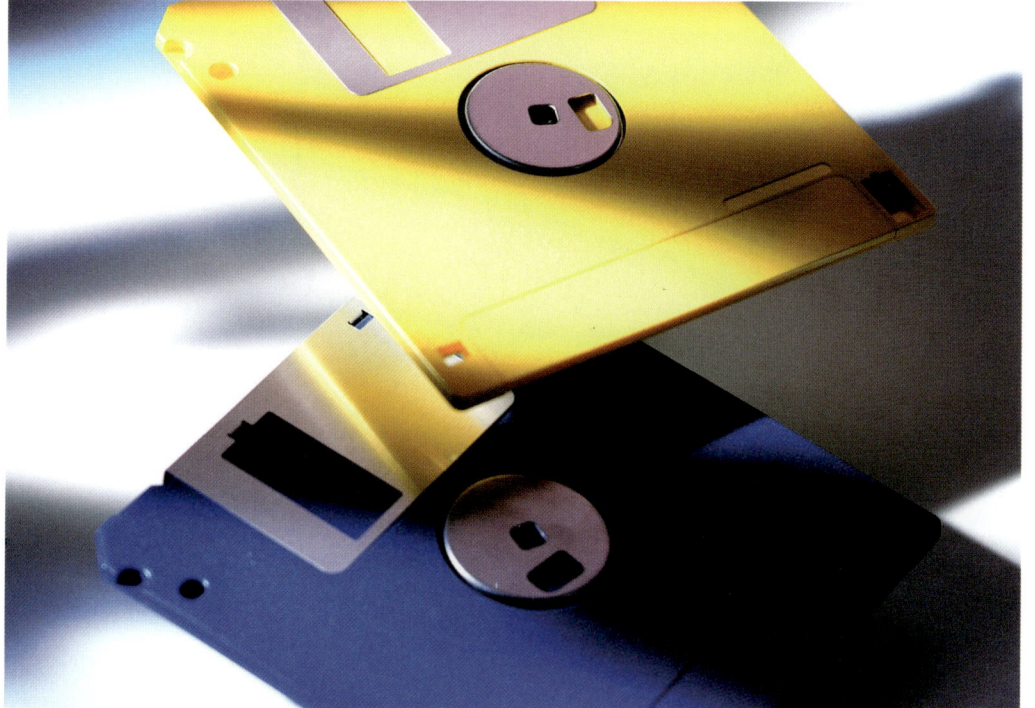

Blue and Orange:

The orange personality is marked by flamboyance and extravagance while the blue folk are mild mannered, quiet and watchful. Yet, because of its dynamic interplay, this relationship can actually be very satisfying for both the partners. The blue person can teach self control to the orange who may be offended by it initially but sharp as they are, they will soon adapt themselves to it. They would realize that self control suits them and helps them achieve what they want. The orange person, on the other hand, has the blue person totally bewitched. The vivacious orange person will teach the blue to enjoy life with gay abandon. The dictum of opposites attracting is most applicable here and neither of the two will ever dislike the balance they can achieve despite their polarity.

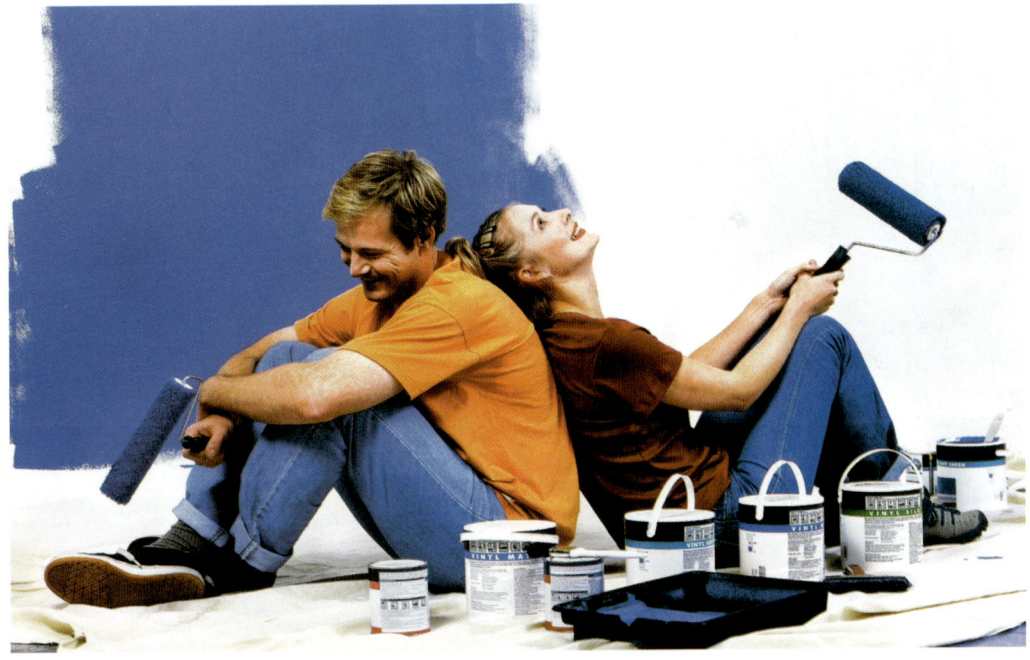

Blue and Pink:

This is a peculiar combination that has just as many chances of working out as it has of not working out. This is because both the pink and blue folk have one strong need in common and that is their necessity to be sheltered and protected always. Both may strive to comfort and support each other but might end up feeling the vacuum of protection themselves. The pink personality is an out- and- out romantic, finding all the bliss in the world, in the arms of an expressive partner and the blue personality is also similar only a bit restrained, initially. However, when this person lets go, there is no looking back.

Brown and Blue:

This combination is an unconventional one but works out effectively for both the partners. The brown personality is very stable and

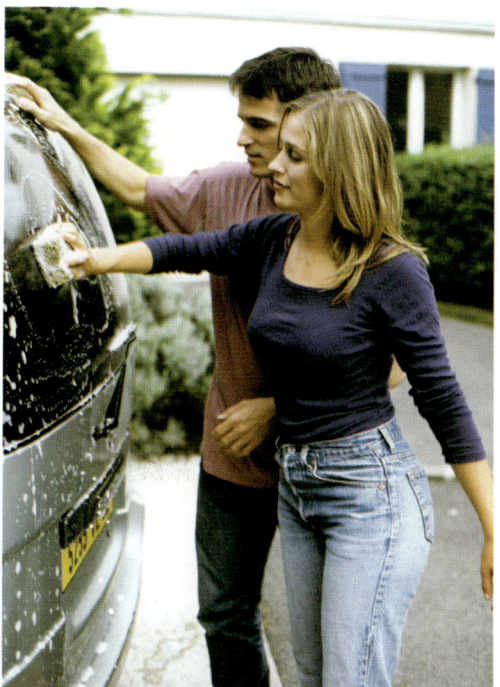
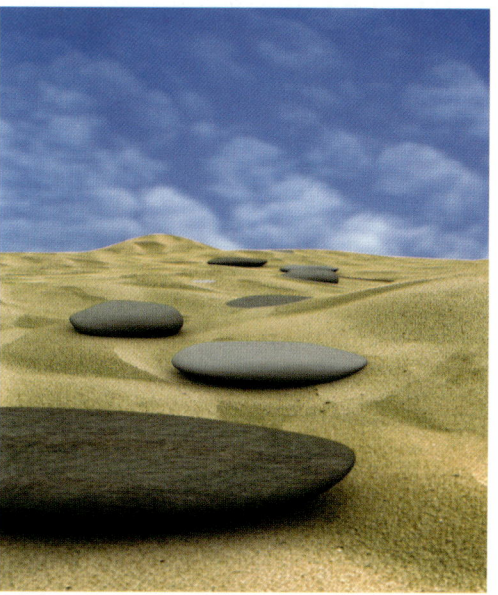

principled and these are the very traits that the blue person finds alluring in a brown person. The dependability of the blue person appeals most to the brown person. The flip side in this relationship could be the fact that while for the blue person, love is a serious matter of the heart that can never be given a secondary position, the brown person has a tendency to equate love with other emotions. This leaves the blue person baffled. This trait has a very negative effect as the brown person fails to instill a sense of priority in the blue folk. It upsets the brown person yet it is not an impossible relationship if both partners are willing to put in a lot of extra effort.

Blue and Black:

Blue and black is a combination which is either well accepted or totally discarded. Same is applicable to people who like black and blue. What works in favour of this couple is the fact that both the blue and black persons

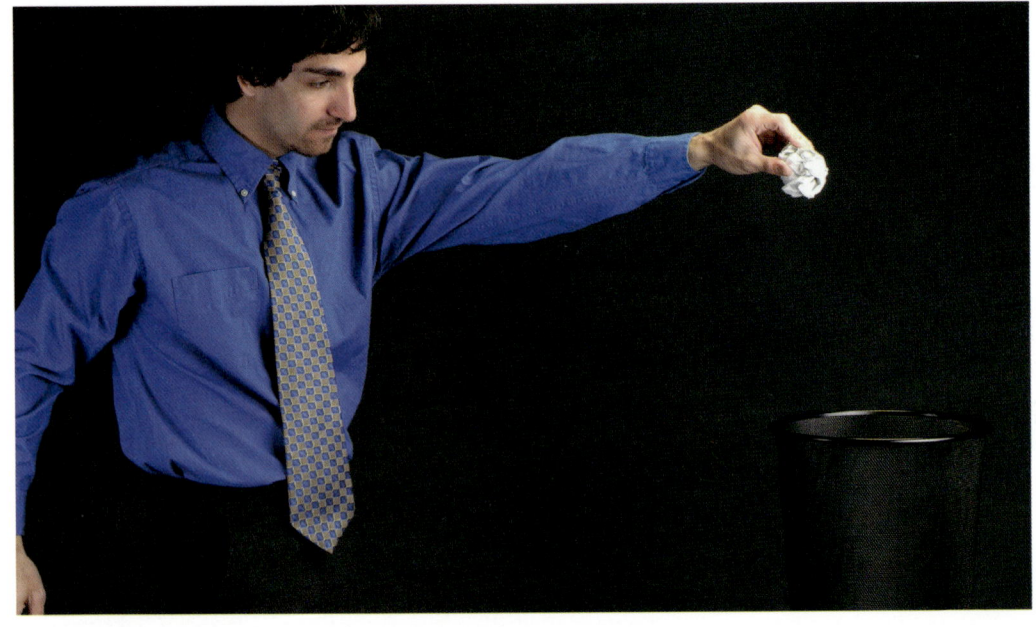

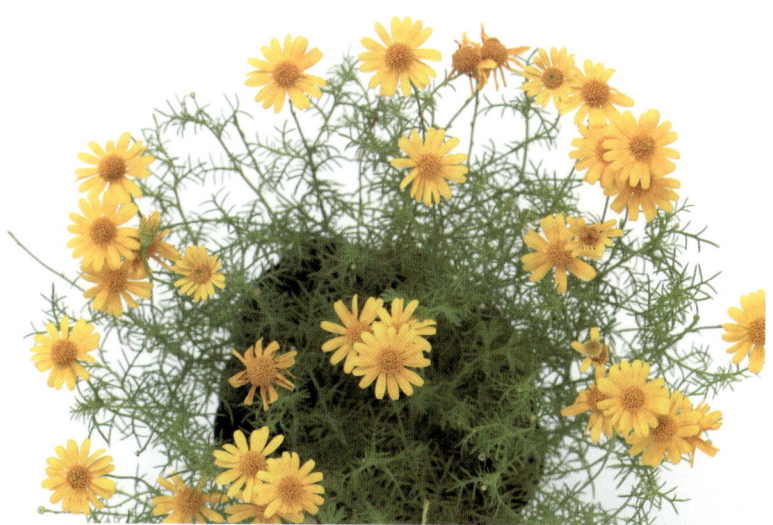

are seeking emotional security. This is the real foundation of love which they find in each other and that results in immense contentment for both. Love is the sensuality of listening to soft music on a moonlit night both to the black and blue personalities. The place where they differ is that the blue personality likes calm and peaceful things while the black folk tend to hunt for greater experiences in life, which could include unravelling the occult. With a complete understanding of each other's intrinsic traits, a beautiful relationship is inevitable.

Green and Yellow:

The green person can be typified as an intellectual. In his/her spare time he reads endlessly and keeps him/herself abreast of all that is going on around. The yellow personality, with all the zest and enthusiasm stimulates the green and actually helps him/her to apply all the knowledge in practical situations. The yellow person is almost fatally attracted to the green personality and these two personalities can be and mostly are each other's best friends as well. A great relationship that can easily culminate in a satisfying marriage.

Green and Orange:

This is a relationship that can either assume epic proportions or not work at all. The green person cannot help being dazzled by the vibrant and attention grabbing orange folk while the orange person easily falls for the pink person who can reach out to their inner selves, penetrating through their flamboyant exterior. Each complements the other in what he/she lacks and desires, all due to the magnetic attraction between the two.

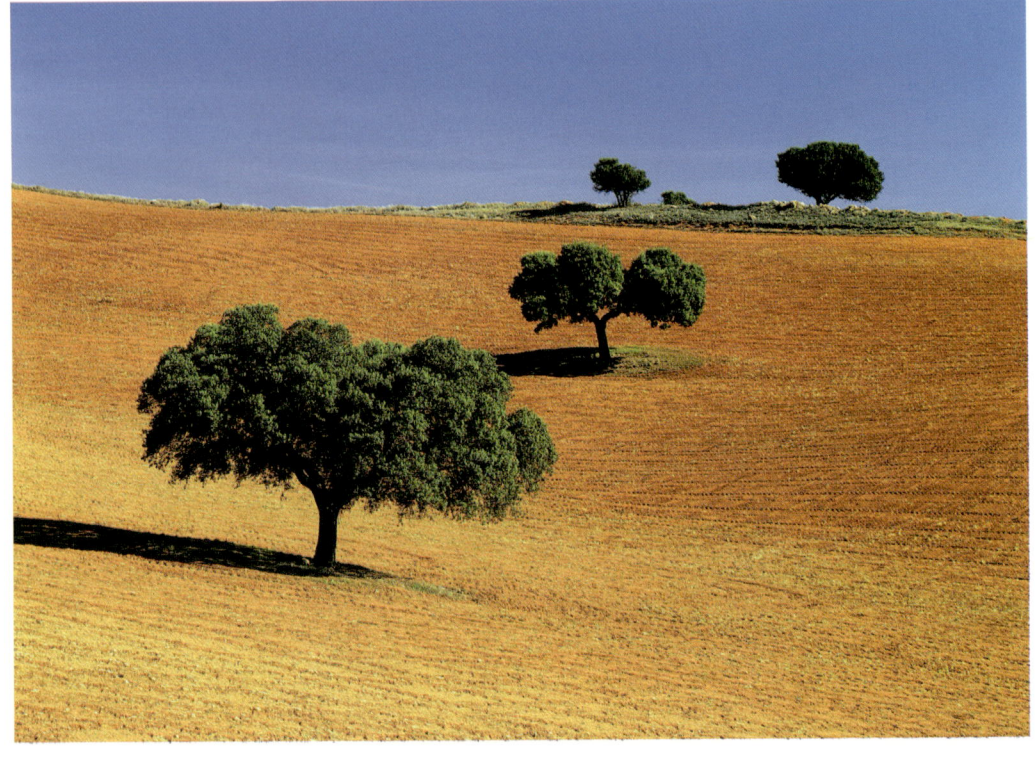

Green and Pink:

The green person is generous and compassionate without restraint. The pink people are just as willing to give all of themselves to a relationship which makes their life meaningful and supersaturated in love. Both being of a mild disposition, there is no friction in the love nest that the green and pink folk set out to make. Sometimes, the stubborn streak in the green person might bother the partner but the pink person has abundant reserves of patience that will ensure that despite the rare instances of obstinacy from the green person, the relationship works out smoothly.

Green and Brown:

The green folk are peace loving and as long as everything around them is in harmony, they are a contented lot. The brown people have a similar approach to life. Both love their home and hearth and will do anything to ensure that everyone in the family is well looked after. This partnership will pave a path for an organisation that will work for a charitable cause or for the underprivileged. A relationship that might lack passion and fervour, yet is stable.

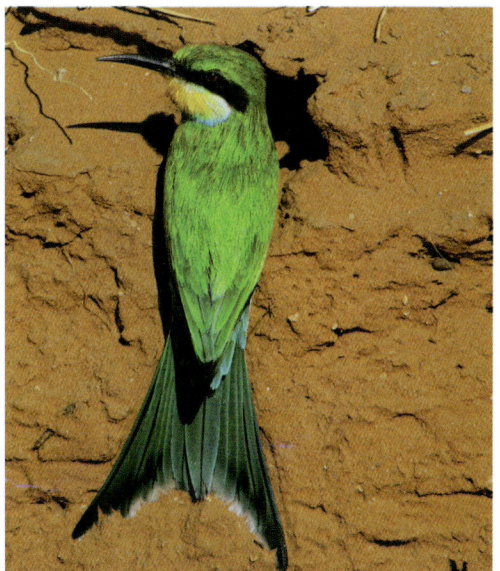

Green and Black:

The green and black personalities are both connoisseurs in their own right. Both have a keen eye for a masterpiece in stone or a beautiful composition. Even exquisite gastronomical delights have a great appeal. Chances are that these two personalities might bump into each other at an exhibition or a wine-tasting party. This very trait keeps the two together. If at all there is a conflict, it is over the black person's lust for adventure of any kind. The green person loves the familiarity of a known environment. However, if the two adopt a mid path, they can enjoy great moments of togetherness.

Yellow and Orange:

The yellow and orange people are a stimulated lot: mentally, emotionally and physically. They look for the same qualities in their partner or else they tire out quite fast and move on without a second thought. This relationship will have all the requisites of a real romance: intense arguments, loads of skirmishes, parting and reconciliation at frequent intervals. Yet at the core of their relationship, will be the sameness that will ensure a hearty and robust life of togetherness.

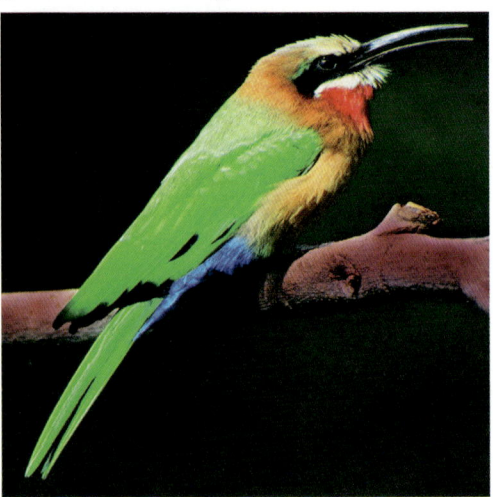

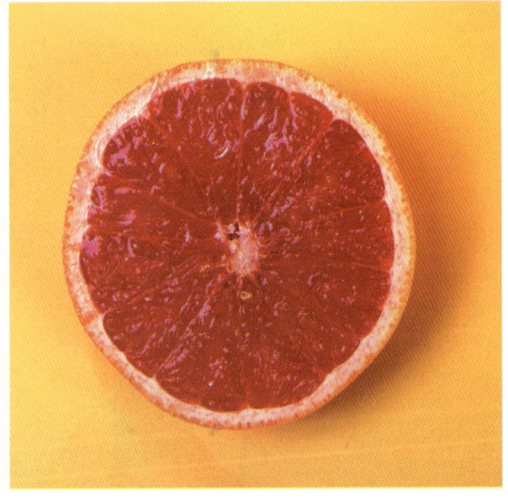

Colour Compatibility

Yellow and Pink:

This relationship is best described as quirky. The yellow person is full of curiosity and experimentation. The pink folk, on the other hand, are happy to remain in known surroundings and if possible would love to retreat to places they have known as children. The two have nothing in common but the pink personality can happily take the backseat and allow the yellow partner to take the lead. This suits the yellow folk well as they love being the centre of attraction, at a party or in a relationship. The yellow person remains in the limelight and the pink person refracts all attention on the partner. Though idiosyncratic, a balance can be struck to make this relationship last.

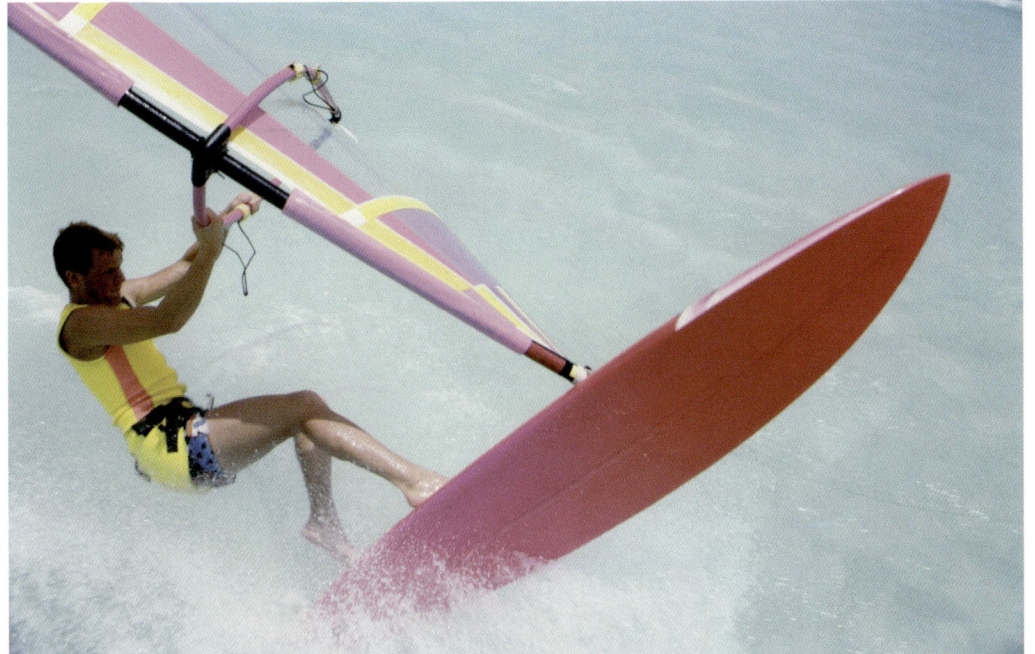

Yellow and Brown:

The yellow personality thrives on the intrigue factor. The more captivating a person is with his/her air of mystery, the more is a yellow person allured. The brown folk, are like an open book with nothing to hide. This can cause a problem in the brown and yellow relationship. The yellow person is freedom-loving and unconventional while the brown person is rooted in the familiarity of things around him/her. The only thing that could bring this couple together is the love for travel and outdoors which both have in plenty. This common interest, if strong enough, can enable the yellow and brown couple to achieve a state of bliss together.

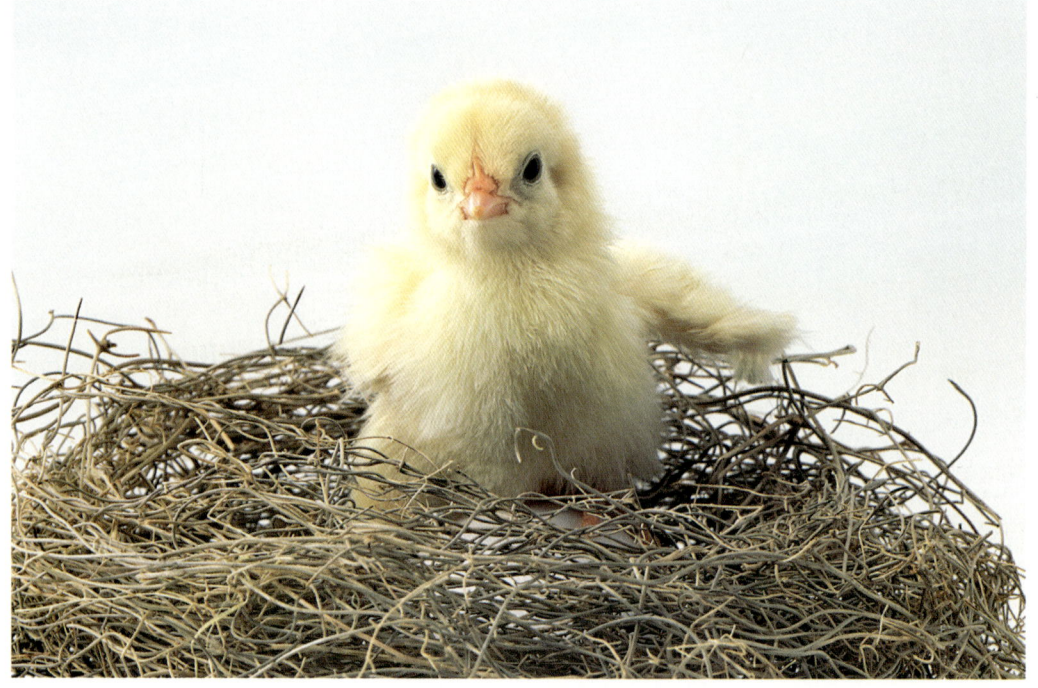

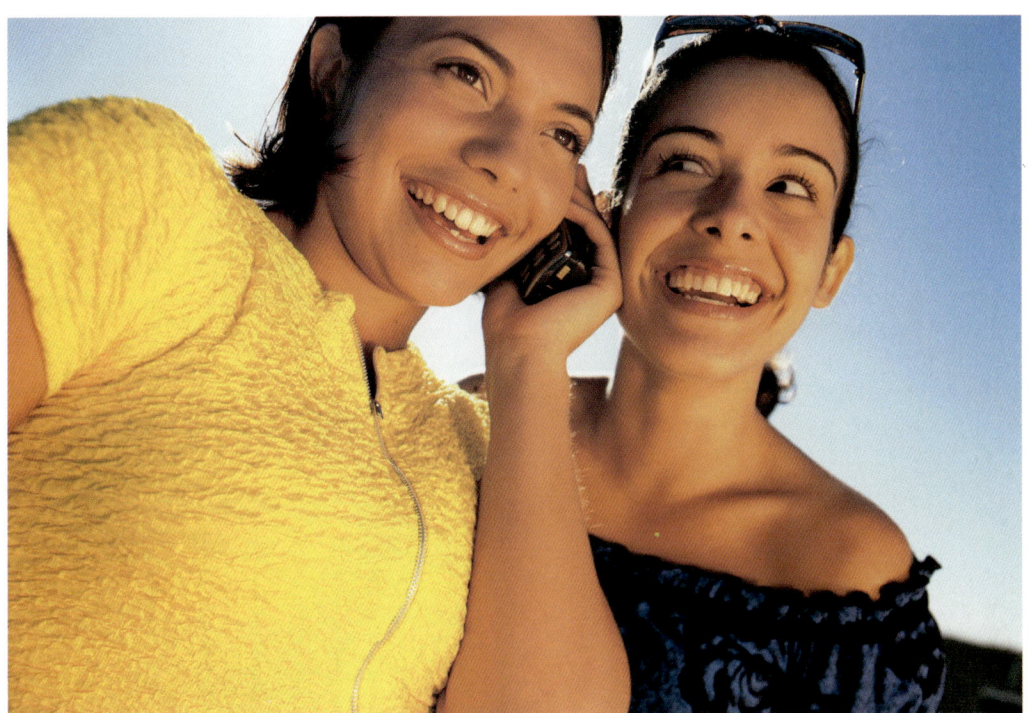

Yellow and Black:

This relationship has the potential to lead to a good and fulfilling romance. The yellow person loves the thought of travelling across the world with a good story to tell at the end of each journey. The black person also echoes the same thought, all set to note down every detail. The black individual is dignified and stately who is impressed by the extra ordinary wit and humour of the yellow person. Both are candid and worry least over being politically- correct. It is this trait that sets them apart from the crowd and makes them love each other even more. A great relationship that can easily translate into marital bliss for both.

Orange and Pink:

The orange person loves the spotlight and the drama that goes with it to a point they almost consider it their birthright. The pink individual, on the other hand, loves to admire and be in awe of his/her partner. This suits both the people in a relationship. One loves the limelight while the other prefers to sit back and smile at the partner for being the centre of attraction. The only problem that can arise is from the fact that the orange folk love to be kept on their toes where they are constantly stimulated mentally and physically throughout their relationship. This might tire out the pink person who does not enjoy power games, in bed or in life in general. An unusual relationship that may work depending on the dedication of the partners to make it successful.

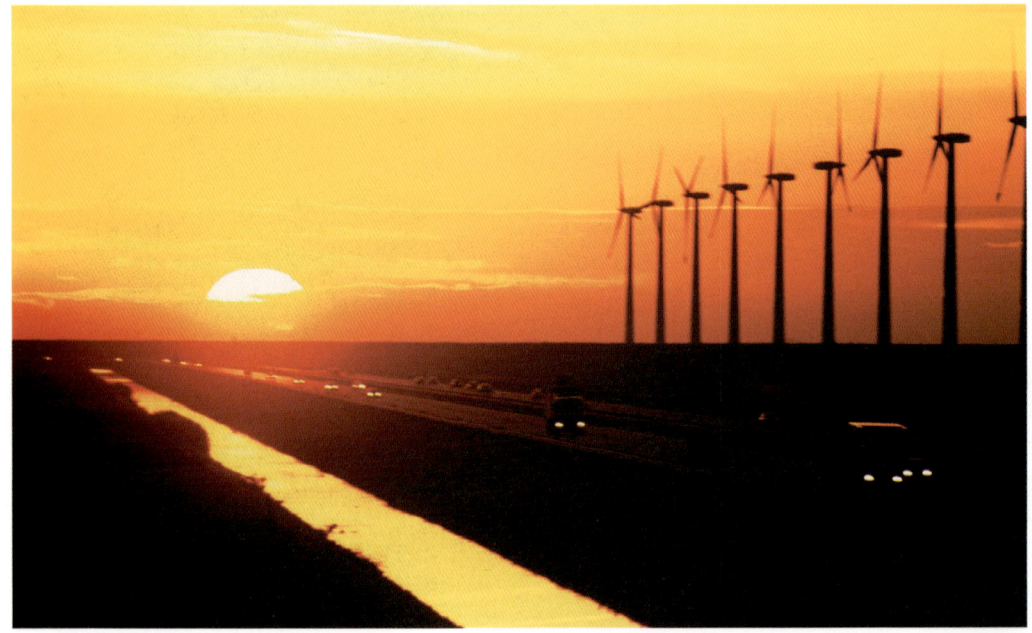

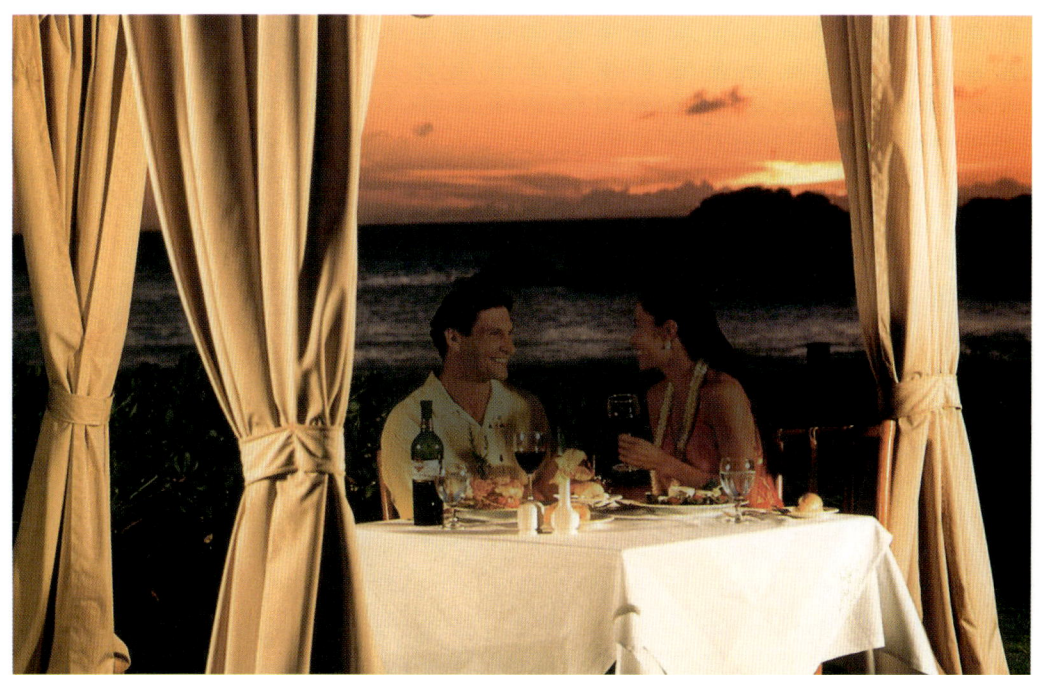

Orange and Brown:

This can be a fairly confusing relationship. The orange person covets the company of those who are intellectual and sincere, the qualities that the brown person possesses. The brown persons on the other hand sometimes need a refreshing change from their humdrum lives and the spunk of the orange personality adds that spice to his/her life. Once the orange person has made up his/her mind about what he/she wants, then there is no looking back. The brown person's sense of commitment, contributes to the relationship. The flip side is that the orange person loves to sensationalise everything from the mundane to the most exciting. The brown person dislikes histrionics of any kind. This is where a conflict may raise its head.

Orange and Black:

The orange person is pretentious and this artificiality, at times, borders on eccentricity. The black personality is sombre and poised. This absolute polarity between the two personality types is what attracts them to each other. As the relationship progresses, the black personality could influence the orange partner to exercise restraint while the orange personality could help the black personality to learn to unwind and revel in the spirit of adventure. This relationship can have the most beautiful moments of their lives provided they can overlook the other's eccentricities.

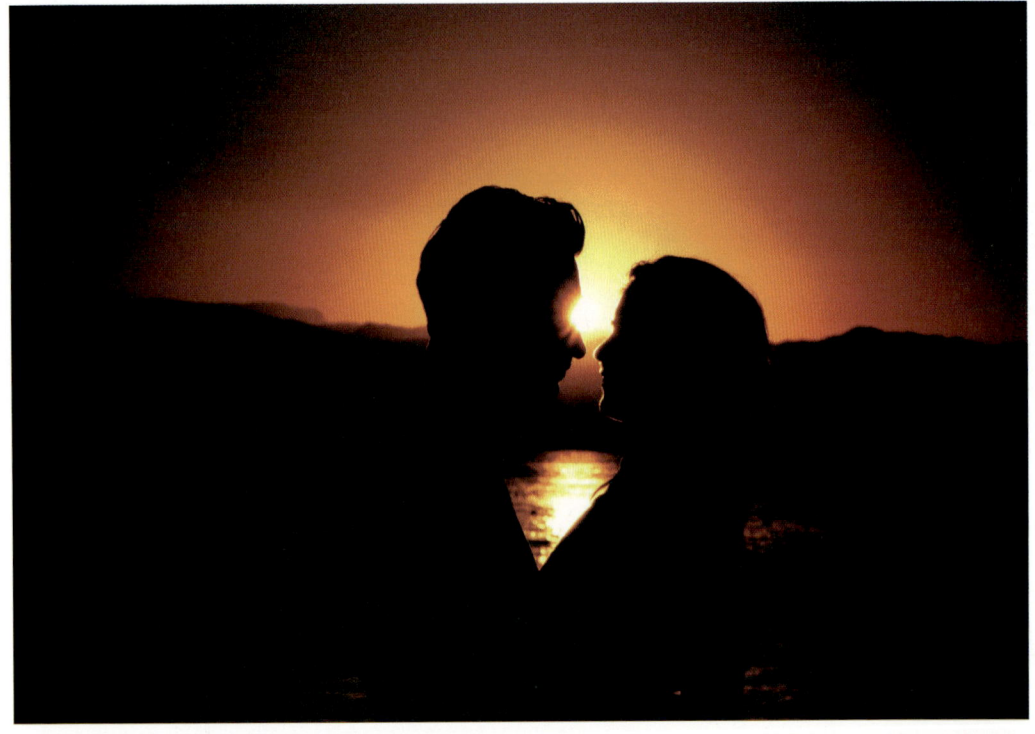

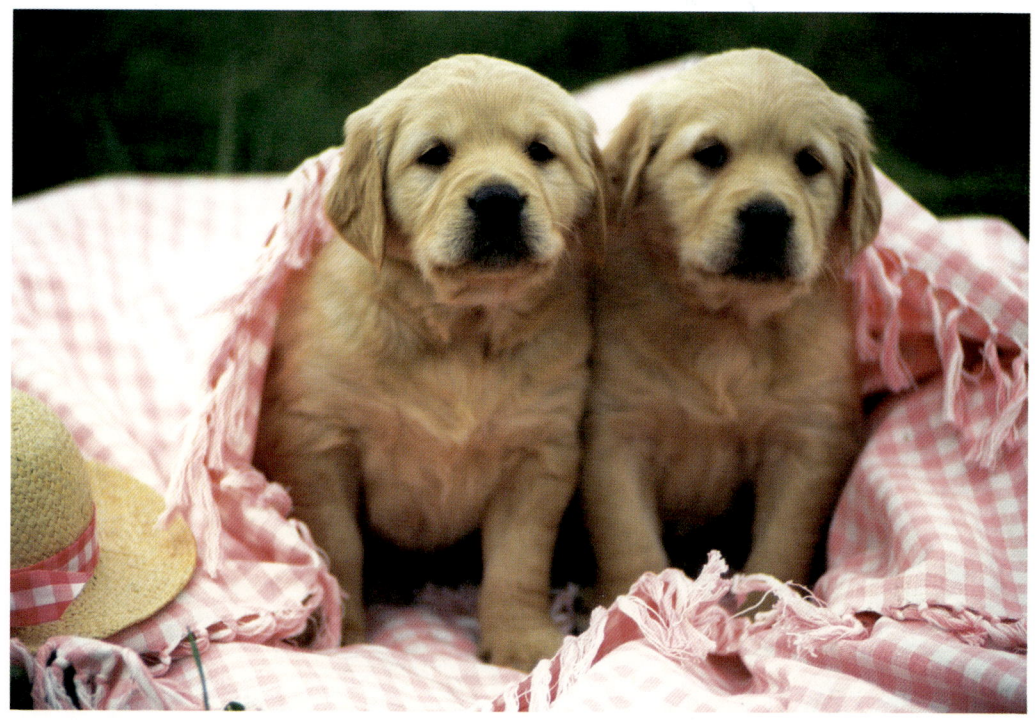

Pink and Brown:

The pink people are a rare breed of romantic dreamers who base everything in their lives on their dreams. The brown folk, on the other hand, are a practical lot who strongly believe in the ethical and moralistic values and for whom realism is the base of every assumption. When these two meet they complement each other by filling in the void in the partner's personality. While the pink person brings the much needed romance in the brown person's life, the brown guarantees the warmth and security in a relationship, which the pink person covets most. Overall, a remarkable relationship that spells a successful marriage.

Pink and Black:

The black personality is a leader, a pacesetter who thrives on the radical and the unconventional. Although he/she might appear to be an epitome of poise and dignity, their mind is constantly searching the avant-garde and the eccentric. The pink person on the other hand, are sensitive, benevolent, romantic and keen on devoting themselves to a humanitarian cause. The two have little in common. While the pink person wants security and commitment, the black personality can't bear accountability and that is why the friction begins. It is not an easy relationship by any means. It may work only if the couple is determined to make it so.

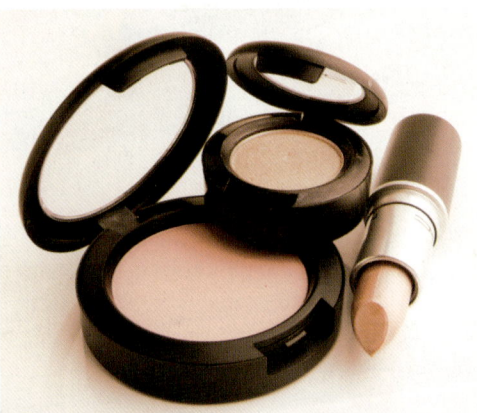

Brown and Black:

This is not an easy relationship to handle. The brown person is very conservative in all that he/she thinks and does while the black person is exactly the opposite: unconventional and progressive. The black person dislikes relinquishing his/her spirit of adventure and general independence while the brown person loves the environs of the home and family where things tend to border on the routine, something that majorly unsettles the black individual. A complex relationship which might need more than just fortitude to make it work.

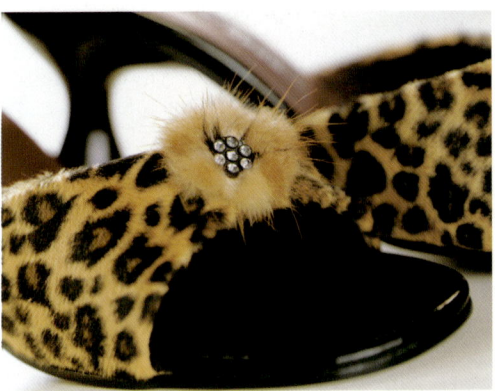

Chapter 6
TOWARDS A HEALTHY AND BEAUTIFUL RELATIONSHIP

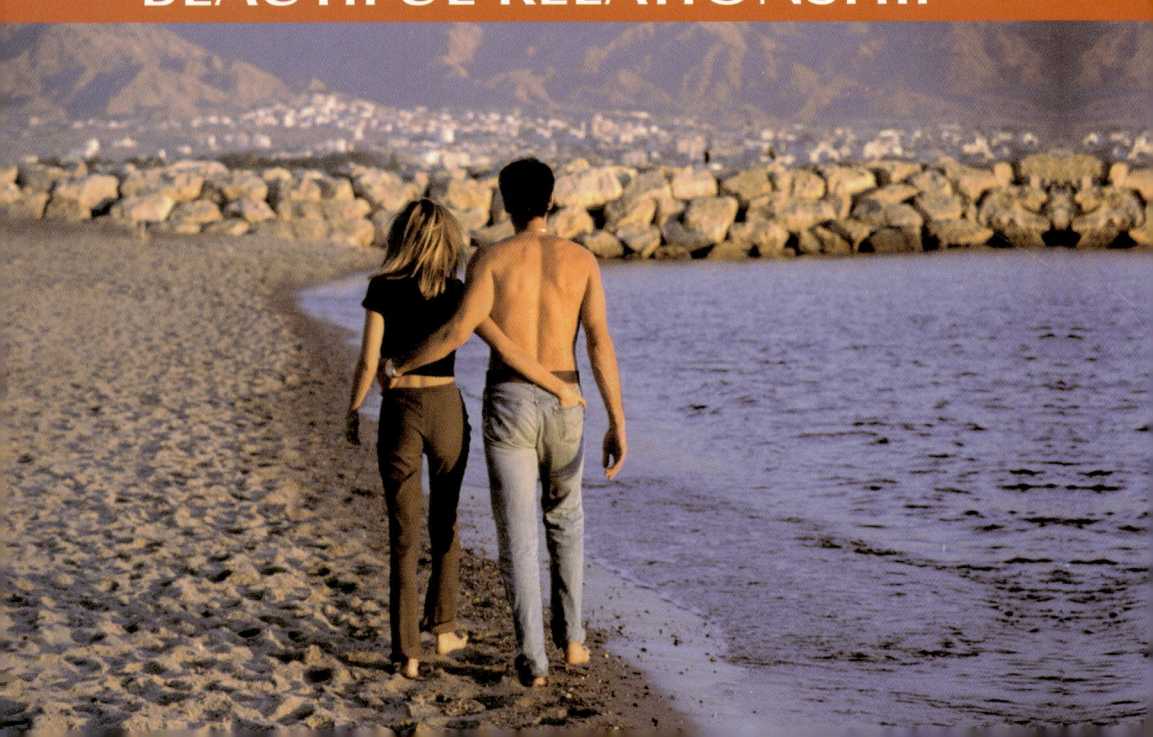

Step 1: Discover the joys of communication:

Relationships, like plants, are tender and fragile. They need constant nurturing. Sometimes, after the two have been together for a while, they tend to lose that spark in their relationship, the very foundation on which human bonds are made.

Preserving relationships, whether it is a marriage or a long association between two partners, is a delicate art and very often, people find themselves at a loss as to how to restore a beautiful relationship, gone wrong.

Colours can go a long way in ameliorating a dreary life pattern and restoring the romance that couples had begun with.

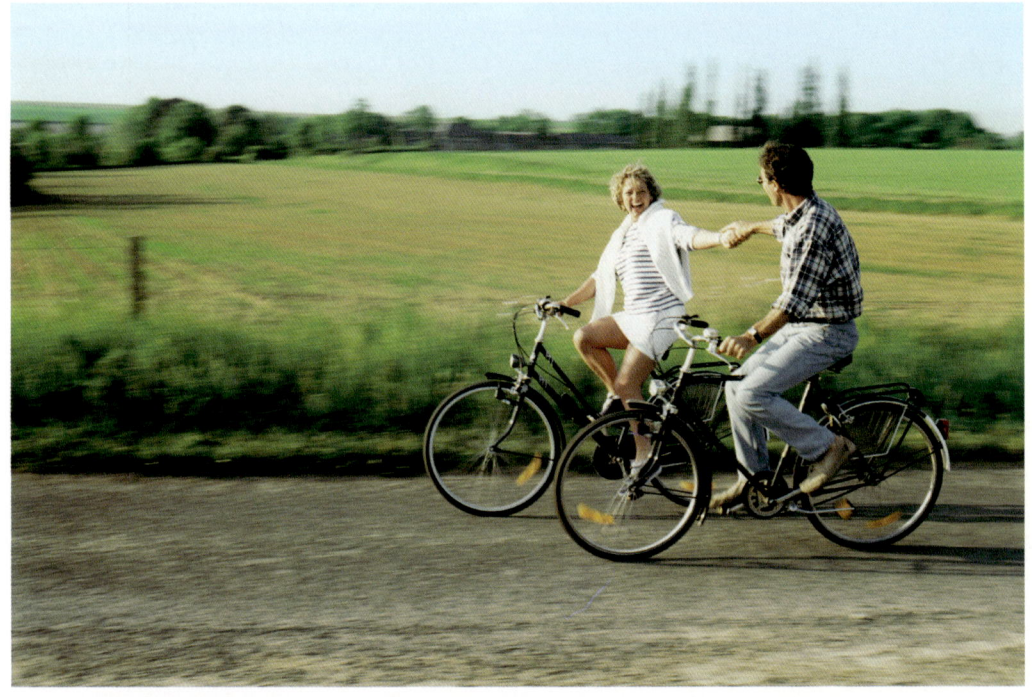

Towards a Healthy and Beautiful Relationship

Communication:

One of the most common relationship problems is the lack of communication. After a certain point, the partners refuse to communicate with each other and begin to lead independent lives. There are also times when one partner might be overtly temperamental, causing stress and anxiety to the other and hurtling a relationship to a disastrous climax.

Blue is the colour that can eliminate communication-related problems in a relationship. The most tranquil colour in nature, it has a calming effect on the mind and body. In some cultures, blue is considered to keep evil spirits at bay and this applies to

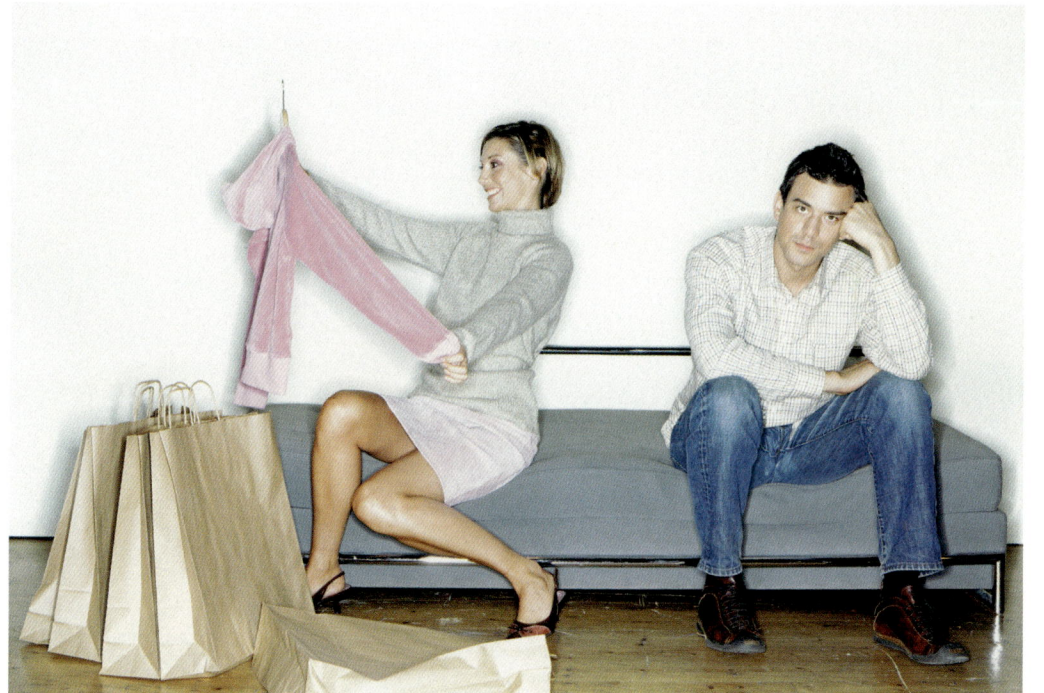

relationships as well. When used correctly, blue can diminish all unpleasantness in a relationship.

Using blue in the bedroom enhances the ability to communicate. Even a hot tempered person feels peaceful. This is the reason why blue is extensively used the world over in the treatment wards of patients with mental volatility. When doing up the wall, diverse patterns and textures in blue can be incorporated. Reminiscent of water, blue is a very good colour to use in case of insomnia. The lighter tints of blue promote healthy and better quality of sleep.

Blue can be incorporated in a room in the form of carpeting also. If one desires, it can be brought into prominence by using blue upholstery and draperies. The choice of tints

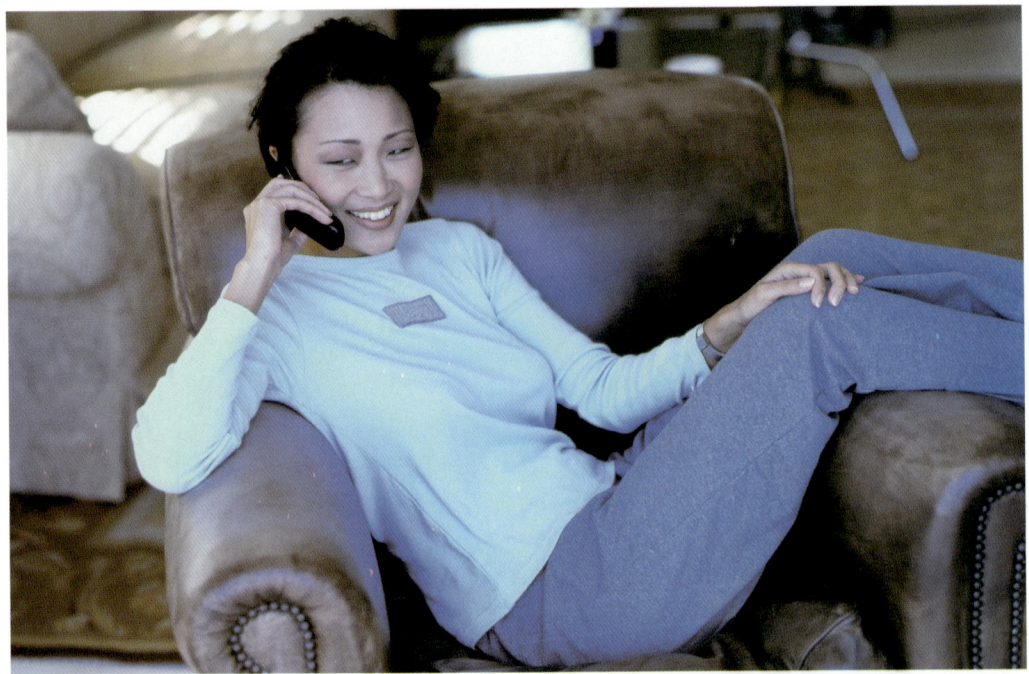

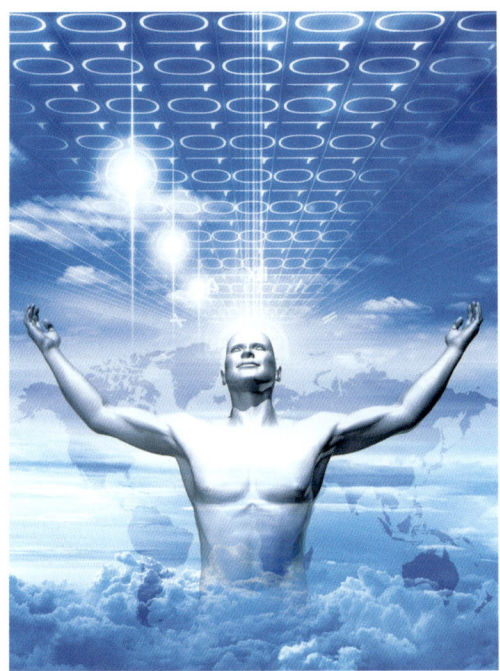

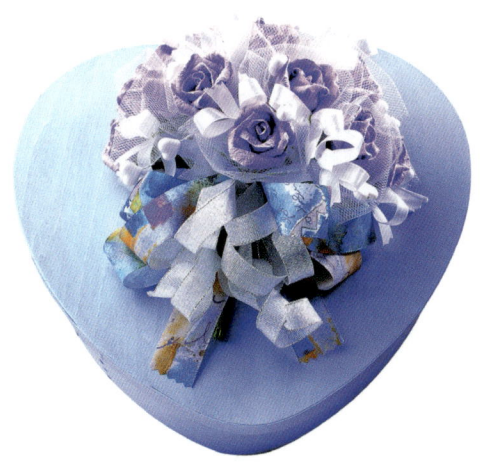

is endless: from teal to aqua, there is always that one special hue of blue that tugs your heart strings.

Blue invokes a trance-like state wherein one's nerves calm down which makes one feel at ease. This enhances the ability of a person to have more comprehensive thoughts and to communicate better. This colour effect can be achieved in a room by lighting a blue bulb, which lends an aura of this colour to the room, making it a haven of peace and tranquillity.

Simply by adding blue flowers to a room or house one can open up channels of communication and bring cheer to the room. There are a variety of blue colours from which one can choose: monkshood, the tall and spiky flowers that are famed for their longevity or sea holly which is such a striking blue that one can meditate upon it endlessly.

In situations where peace and tranquillity need to be brought into a relationship, candles as a medium of colour and cosmic energy

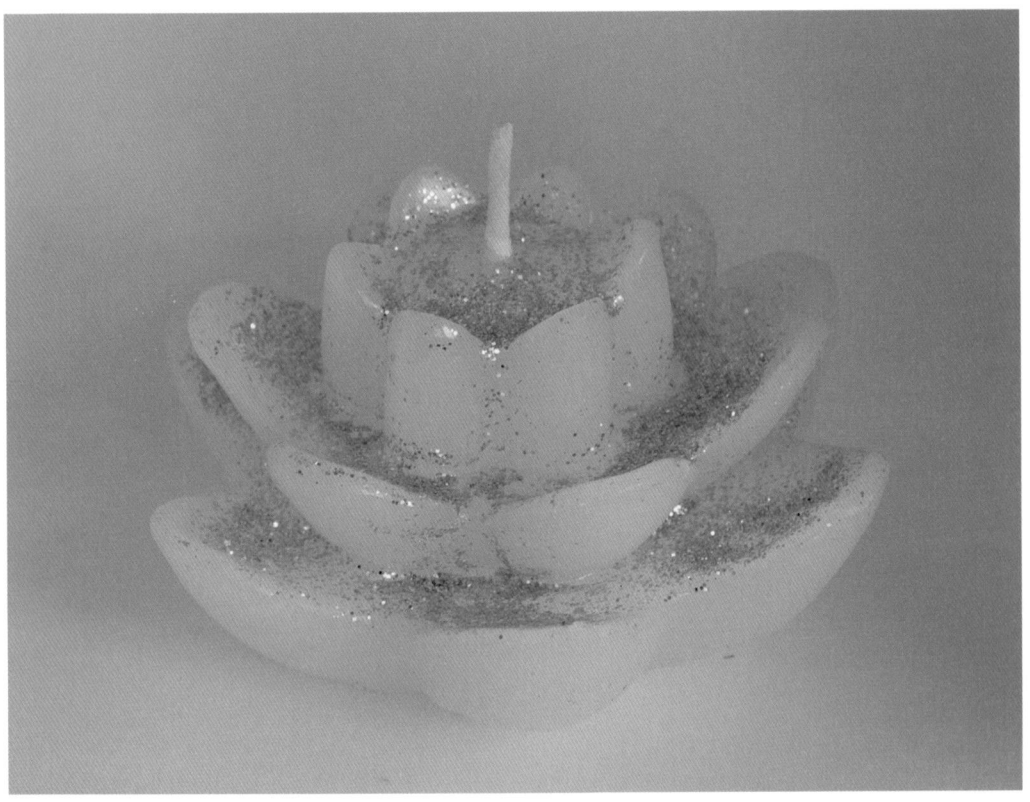

can be used effectively. In this case, light blue candles should be used. These promote understanding, sincerity and open up channels of communication between two people. Ideally, the candles should be lit for at least half an hour daily, once the work for the day is over, in order to recharge the mind and soul.

Eating large portions of blue foods, like blue berries, too works wonders. Being evocative, it promotes hope, fidelity and opens channels of communication. This colour can be meditated upon for its therapeutic qualities or simply adding this colour to one's wardrobe helps.

For the indulgent ones, adding scented oils which correspond to the blue colour like lily of the valley, jasmine, lotus and cedar not only makes bathing a pleasurable experience but also provides the restorative properties of blue.

Another option of incorporating blue in one's life is through colour breathing. The technique is simple and can be practised at any time when one is relaxed and calm, in the morning or before going to sleep. Sit or lie down in a comfortable position and ensure that the body is warm. Then, proceed to breathe in a calm, relaxed way so that the breathing pattern is even. Visualize blue coloured vertical rays descending from heaven towards the body and you are absorbing the rays through your

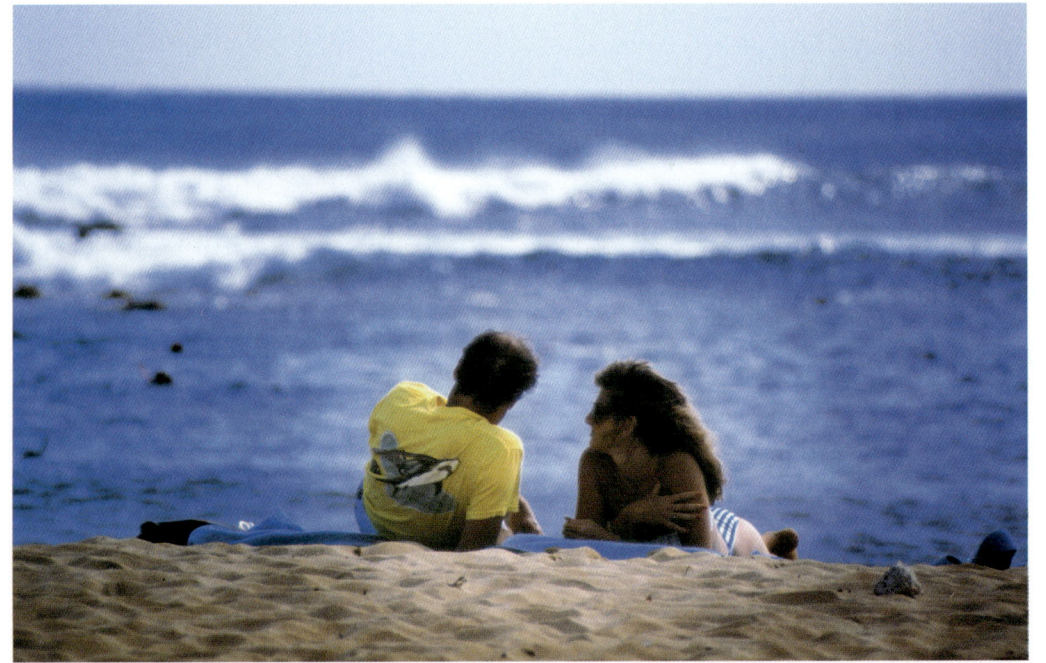

breathing. Picture the blue rays penetrating each part of your body and as you breathe out visualize exhaling orange colour from your body. This exercise should be ideally done for five minutes every day for maximum benefit. It also benefits those suffering from insomnia and women with menstrual problems.

One can listen to blue music that can enhance a person's ability to communicate. Blue music is that which relates to the key of G in a musical spectrum and its calming effects are felt not only on the body but also the mind which is relaxed. In such a composed and calm state every thing else falls into place. Examples of blue music are ' Jesu Joy of Man's Desirings' and ' Air on a G string ' both composed by Bach. Turquoise is another colour which promotes better communication between partners. It blends the hues of blue and green, combining the balance and stability of green with the frankness of blue. It has the pacifying effects of blue as well as the soporific qualities of green. This colour can be incorporated in the form of gemstones, the interiors of a room or worn as a dress by the person to avail its benefits.

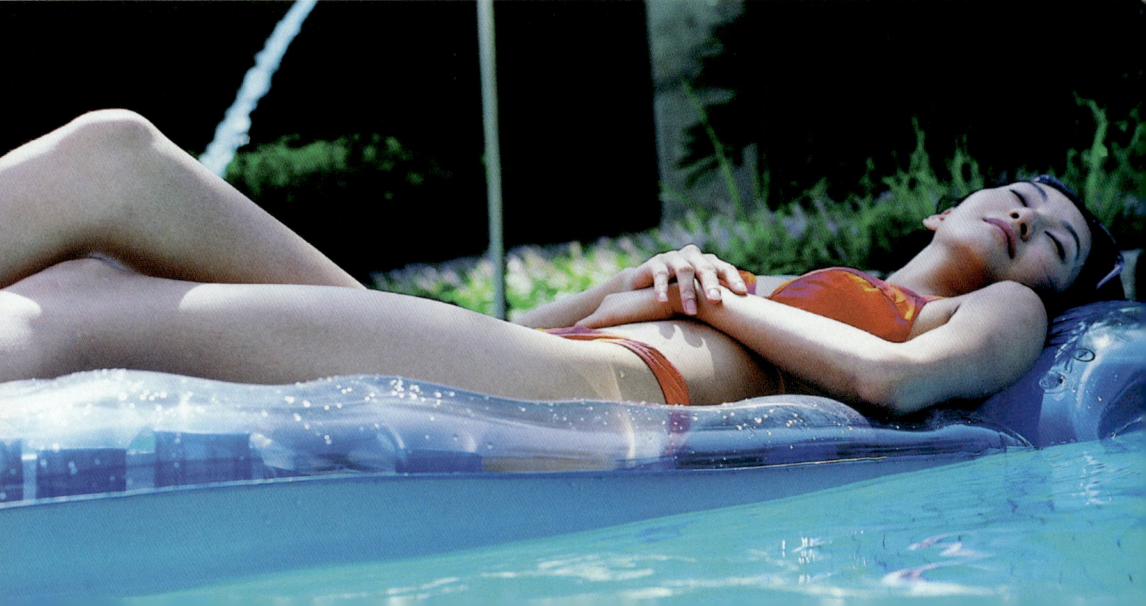

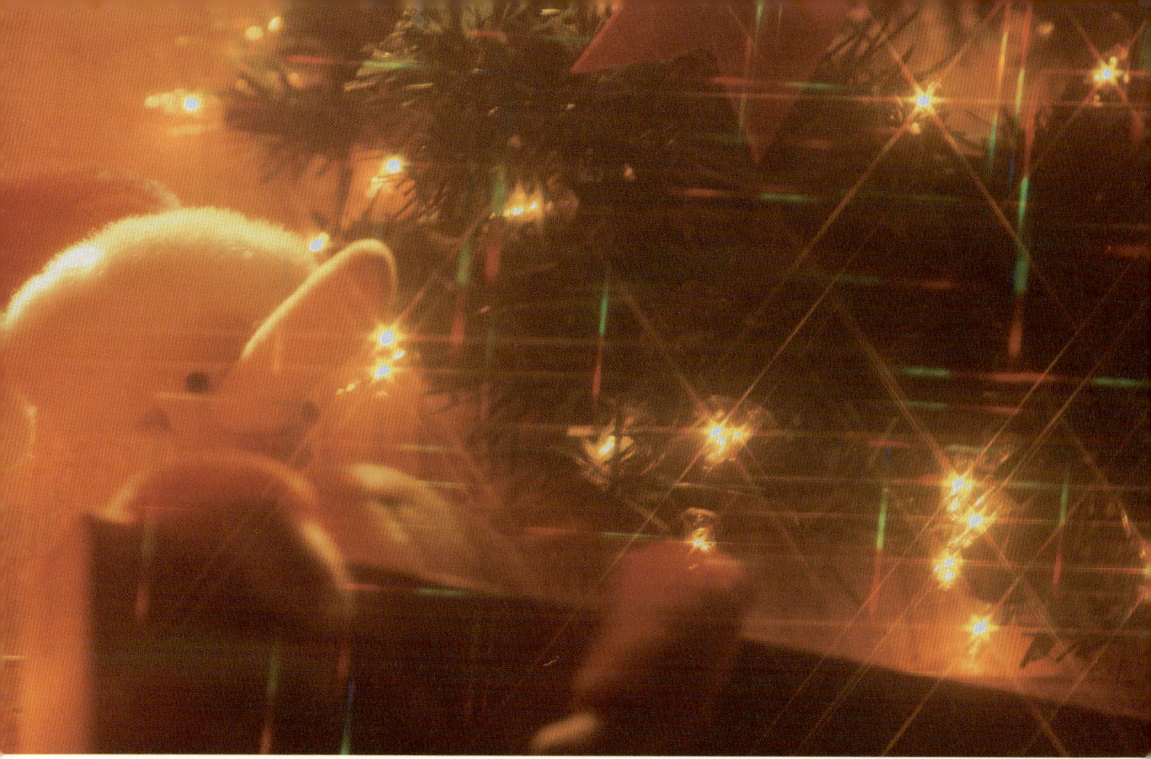

Orange is the happiest colour – Frank Sinatra

Orange is another fantastic colour option to get two people to talk or to open up. Being a mixture of red and yellow, it has the characteristics of both: the vivacity and energy of red and the warmth and good cheer of yellow. Orange increases the blood supply to the brain thus invigorating the body as well as charging the intellect, giving it greater clarity and perspective.

Orange, incorporated in the interiors of a house, brings a sense of exuberance to the environment. It is an ideal colour to use in dining areas, living rooms and passages in the house. Its effects become apparent in very little time. In its pure form, it might be a tad too hot for the bedroom. When used in its various shades and tints or when combined with other colours, it can a whole new meaning to a relationship. Shades like tangerine or melon tend to do exceedingly well in the living or dining areas. If one desires to use orange in a bedroom then a better option is to combine it with cool and earthy hues.

Peach, a derivative of orange is a good colour option if a single colour is to be used. It gives the room an ambience which releases pent up pressure of the mind and body. It promotes affability and enables partners to communicate more freely. Orange works particularly well in tropical climates. If one wishes to create the same cheery atmosphere to the interiors of one's house, then the ideal combination is that of orange with green. This colour scheme adds zest to the environment, bringing nature indoors. Introducing green in the décor proves soothing both for the mind and body by de stressing them.

Orange stands out when combined with shades of blue. Blue and Orange in a room has the dual effect of calming the nerves as well as making one feel warm and protected both essential for better communication. While the orange tones make one feel embalmed in affability, the blue eliminates paranoia and edginess in a person.

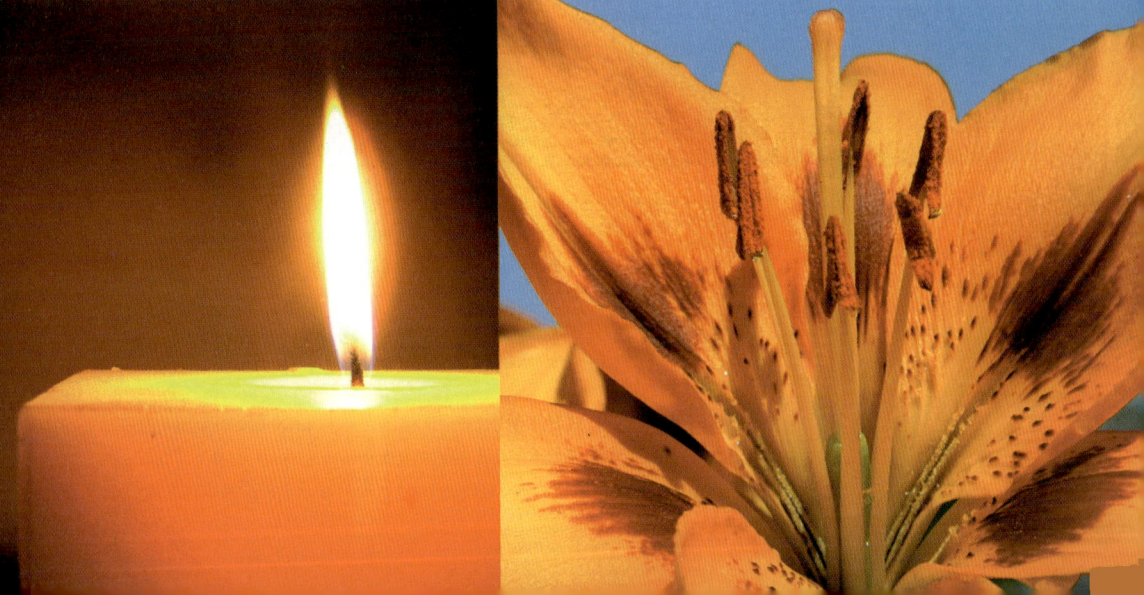

Orange can be added to a room simply by the interplay of light and shade. Orange lamp shades of different hues ranging from terracotta to coral can be placed strategically in a room to create the desired effect: movement and openness.

Another way of including the orange colour in one's daily life is by merging the mundane with the magical and spiritual, by lighting candles which have long been associated with wish fulfillment. Orange candles are ideal for opening communication channels and for replenishing the intellect. Light the candles and focus on what you desire from your relationship. While the candle burns it evokes wish fulfillment and also creates the mood for sitting back and letting go of all the tension and stress within. By the time you are ready to extinguish the candle, you will fell rejuvenated and raring to go.

Moreover, orange colour can be brought into one's life by including orange foods at least in one meal each day. The choices are varied, from the namesake orange to pumpkins and carrots, all one needs to do is to pick out the orange food that they like best and experience

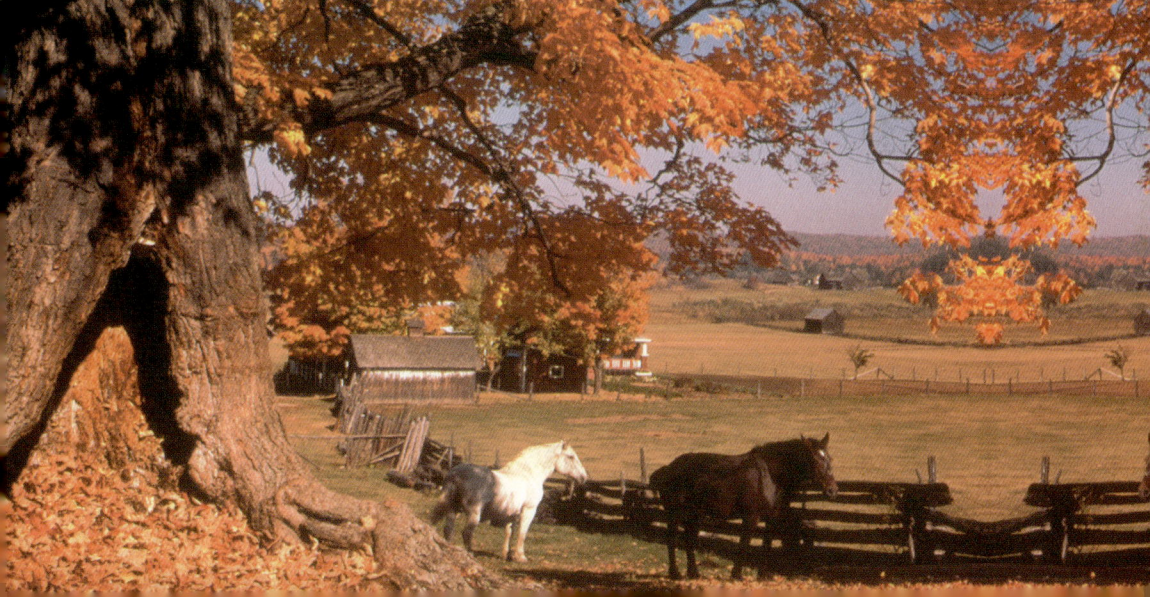

the therapeutic effects of this colour take over.

Reminiscent of autumn, orange evokes feelings of sociability and abundant optimism. This colour can easily be included in one's life by adding it in the wardrobe. Those who wear this citrus colour will not only find it easier to communicate, his/her thoughts to the other person but also evolve on an intellectual level. Orange can be added in one's life by practising breathing in the orange colour. Following nearly the same technique as breathing in blue, create in your mind an image of orange coloured rays seeping into your from the soles of your feet and expanding into every other part of your body as they gradually travel towards the top of your head as you breathe in. As you breathe out, visualize exhaling the blue colour from your body.

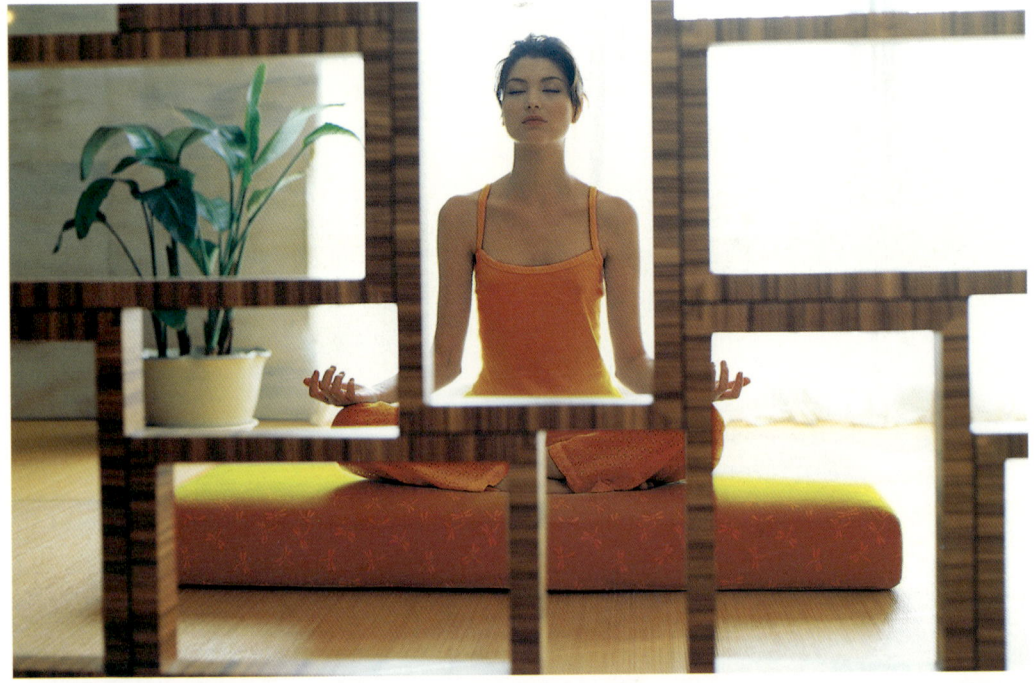

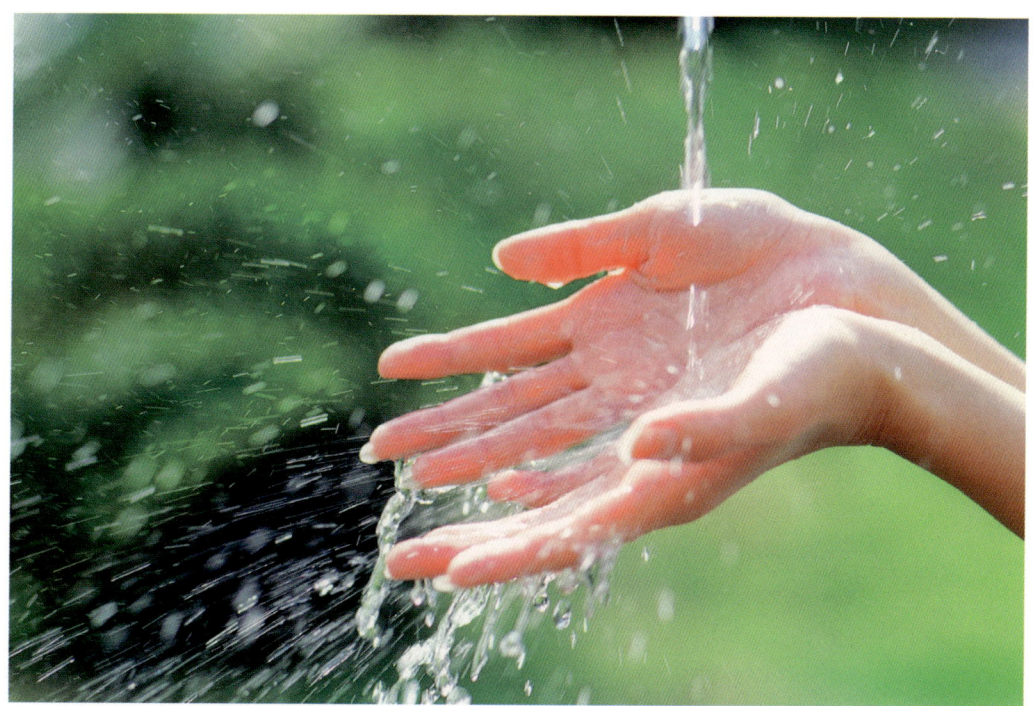

This exercise should ideally be done for five minutes every day for maximum advantage. It is particularly beneficial for treating hyper thyroidism, hypo thyroidism and mental exhaustion.

Music is nature's own therapy. Hearing the gurgling sound of water or the chirping of birds rejuvenates the body and mind.

Orange music adds cheer and vivacity to its environment, expelling negative emotions and charging the atmosphere with positive vibrations. Orange music relates to the key of D in the musical spectrum and some of its fine examples are 'Hallelujah Chorus from The Messiah' by Handel, 'Gloria in excelsis deo' by Vivaldi and 'Waterfall Music' by Paul Warner.

Step 2: The ultimate commitment: Sharing your inner self

Forging a relationship is the beginning of a wonderful journey of two people together. As it progresses leisurely, it unfolds the delight and wonder of being together. However, much as togetherness merges two people into one entity, there are many stumbling blocks on the road to eternal bliss.

Very often, we are in a relationship which is closest to our hearts, we find it difficult

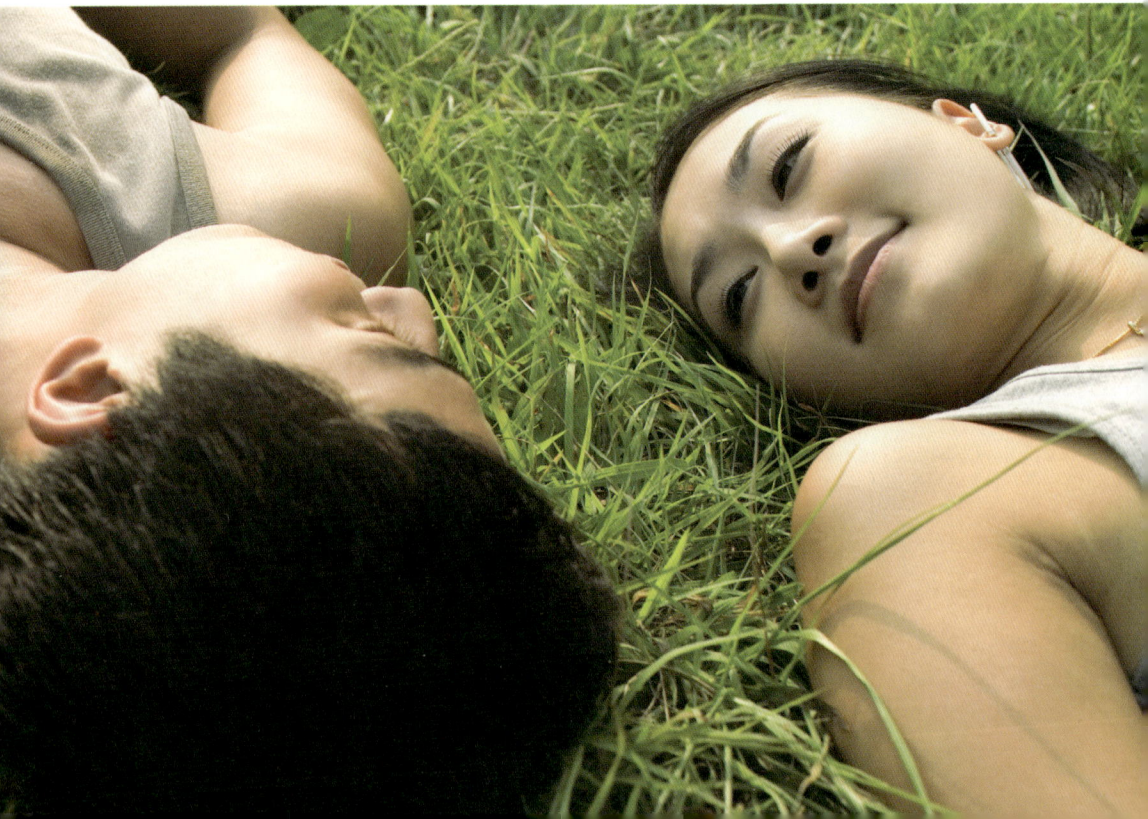

Towards a Healthy and Beautiful Relationship

to open up completely to our partners. In effect, despite giving a lot of ourselves, we are holding a lot back. The real pleasure of a relationship is in absolute surrender, where two people become one in entirety and that is a state not difficult to achieve. With the discreet use of colour, one can surrender oneself completely and that is the ultimate commitment for a satisfying relationship.

The first prerequisite of being able to share oneself with another person is the feeling of being protected, secure and grounded. It is only when a person feels totally at ease within, that his ability to give her/himself becomes enhanced. This can be accomplished by using all shades of brown.

Symbolic of the earth, brown represents the home and hearth, denoting a happy family. People who choose brown over other colours are considered reliable, responsible and sincere. Brown is known to be very effective in dispelling mental depression and offering a sense of stability, thereby enabling one to let go of the guardedness.

Brown also helps chase away indecisiveness and increases concentration levels of the mind. This colour can easily be adapted into one's daily wardrobe since it is an unobtrusive colour, which particularly finds favour with men who consider it is resilient and a rugged hue.

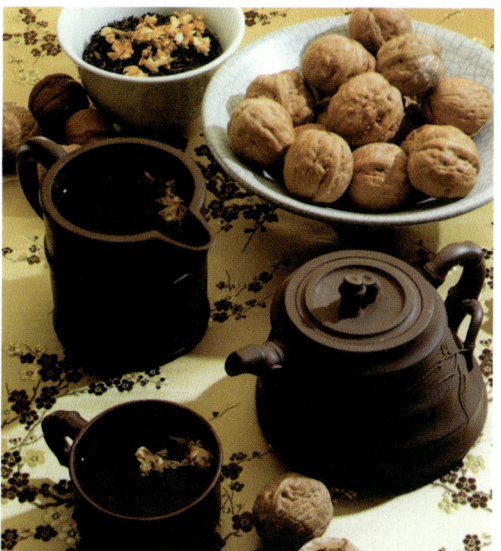

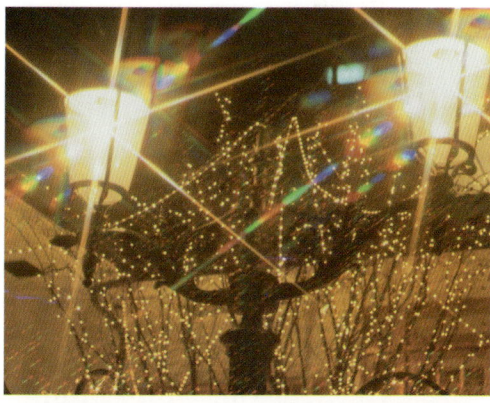

As a colour, brown is considered a neutral shade, which means that it can favorably be combined, with various other colours to create varying moods and convey different messages.

Brown combines well with yellow and lends a natural and comfortable feel. When wearing this combination, you will reach a new comfort level which will make it easier for you to connect with your partner and share all facets of your personality.

Another combination that is very appealing to the men folk is brown and blue. It fuses the earthiness of brown with the calm and relaxed feeling of blue, creating a very cool image of the wearer. This ensures that those around him/her cannot help but let go of his/her guard. It also gives greater insight which enables the person to delve deep into the partner's true self.

The colour of wood, brown can be effectively incorporated in one's interiors to create a feeling of comfort and stability within the home environs. This helps one to trust the partner more easily and thereby share every part of his/her personality with a lot more frankness and confidence.

This assurance evoking colour is part of every room in every house but the trick lies in using it skillfully. While the paler shades of brown add a feeling of cosiness and well-being, which

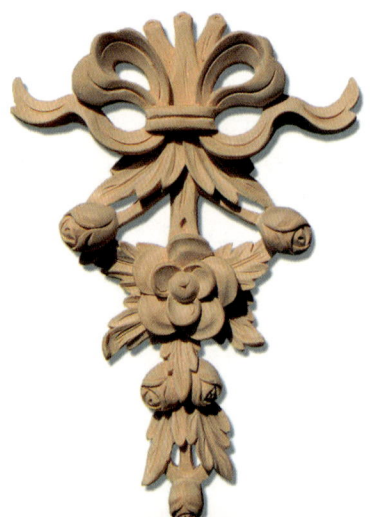

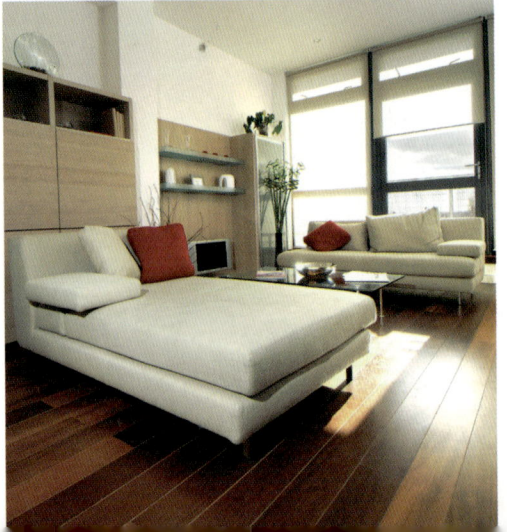

is just what the two people need, in order to share their most intimate selves with the other. In dry climates, the amalgamation of brown with muted reds works best since it absorbs glare and softens a parched looking room.

A lot of people find brown to be a supportive colour that makes them feel more at ease to be able to convey all that they feel or think, no matter how radical or personal.

Most people find colouring their walls in any shade other than white a bit out of place. For such people, the solution is simple; use a painting that has predominant tones of brown in it to add the earthiness of a brown-based colour theme to the interiors of a room. Some classic paintings, reproductions of which are accessible, done in overlaying shades include Paul Cezanne's 'The Card Players', Henri Matisse's 'Reading woman with a Parasol'.

There is also the option of getting in touch with one's inner consciousness by painting a canvas oneself in the preferred shades of brown and then hung to be both admired for its originality as well as the healing it offers.

Tones of the brown colour can be found in various scents like cherry, cloves, lilac to name some. They can be found in over-the –counter products like shampoos, body lotions and bath oils which can all be used to absorb the curative properties of brown. Oil of clove not only causes one to feel comforted and secure but also allows the transformation and renewal of ideas by releasing inhibited energies trapped within the body. Clove, in particular, can be found in the form of incense and the smoke produced thus is said to be aphrodisiacal in nature as well as helps in dispelling the negativity in the area where it is burnt.

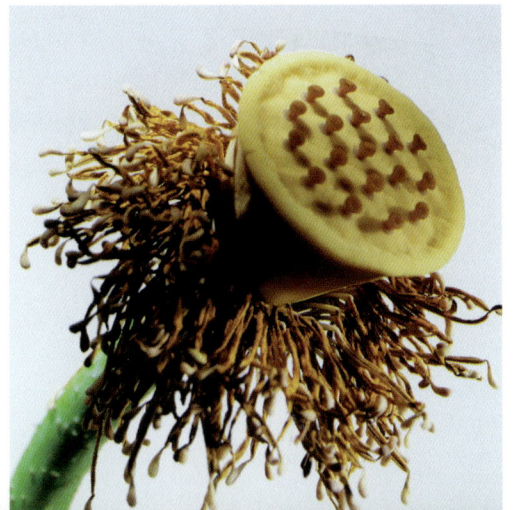

Myrrh, another scent that corresponds to brown, was an indispensable component used in the embalming process by the ancient Egyptians. This fragrance, much like brown, is considered very effective in making one feel grounded and in harmonizing the innermost suppressed emotions of a person, thus

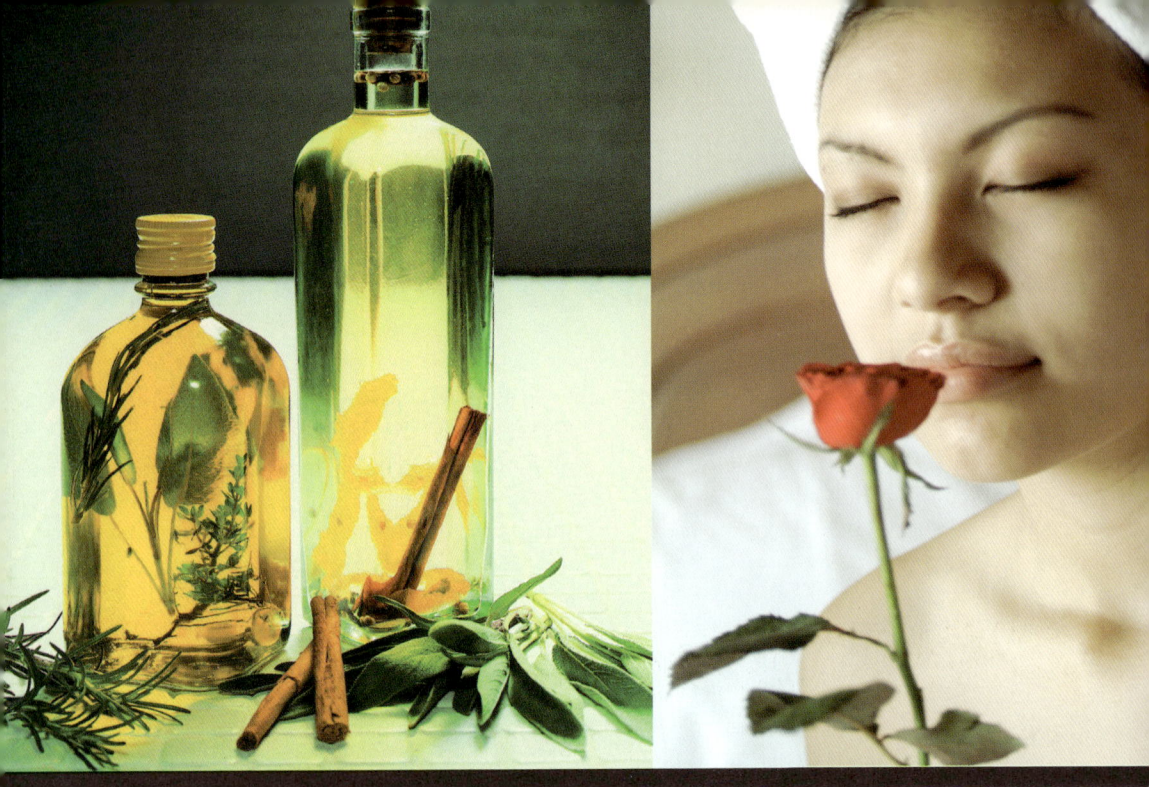

nourishing the soul as well.

Yet another fragrance corresponding to brown is Eagle wood. This scent is found in most parts of Japan where it is an essential component of high-end incense and in Tibetan medicine where it is used to allay melancholy. This scent makes one feel contented and protected, promoting real intimacy.

Brown can be infused in the body by consuming brown coloured foods and what better food than chocolate, a universal favourite. Chocolate contains stimulants like caffeine, theobromine and phenylethylamine, all which contribute to giving one a sense of well-being. Chocolates are not considered the most luxuriant form of therapy for nothing.

One can indulge in this decadent 'comfort-food' either by experimenting with home made chocolate or by indulging in the best

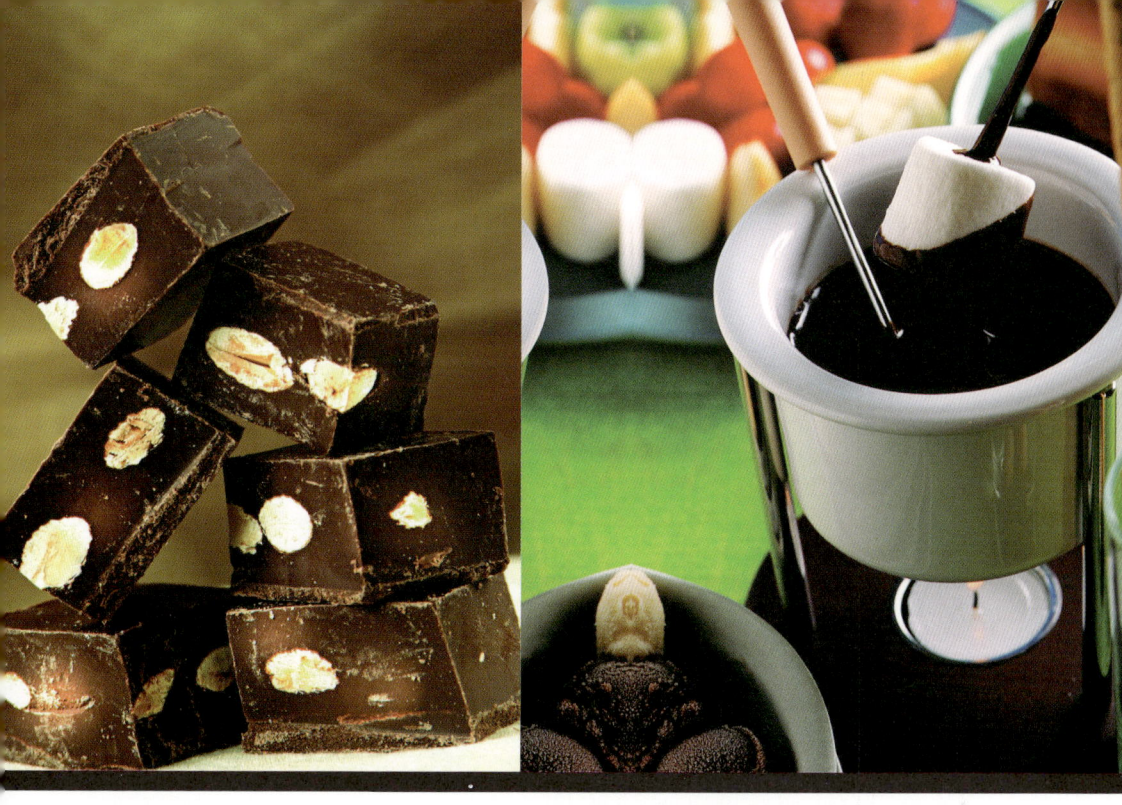

chocolates from around the world that include names like Amadei, Felchin, Marcolini, Lindt, Valrhona and many others which leave the person desiring for more.

CHILLI HOT CHOCOLATE
(Just the way the Mayans had it)
Ingredients:
- 2 ½ cups water
- 1 Chilli pepper slit (de-seeded)
- 6 cups milk
- 1 vanilla bean (slit lengthwise)
- 2 cinnamon sticks
- 1 bar dark chocolate
- Sugar to taste

Method:
In a pan, boil the water and add the slit chilli.

Cook till the water is reduced by half, then drain the chilli and keep the water aside.. In another pan, add the vanilla and cinnamon to the milk and simmer for a few minutes, then add the chocolate bar (broken into medium size pieces) and the sugar.

Whisk till the mixture becomes homogeneous. Remove from the flame. Remove the vanilla and cinnamon and add the chilli little at a time till the hot chocolate acquired a spicy aftertaste. Serve hot.

Step 3: Merging spiritually

Love is not simply being each other's support system alone. It is not about finding one's best friend in a partner. Love is the emotion that truly touches one's heart, body and soul. It is true love when it penetrates from the heart into the soul, merging two people in a unique oneness. Love is what makes the heart swell with emotion and the soul feel comforted and enveloped in a hazy mist of reverence.

To be able to find true love and remain connected to it, implies constant nurturing of the bond between two people that ties their heart and soul together. It means remaining in the trance-like togetherness which can accomplished with an abundance of love in the heart and a little assistance from the colours.

"I think it pissed God off if you walk by the colour purple in a field somewhere and don't notice it"

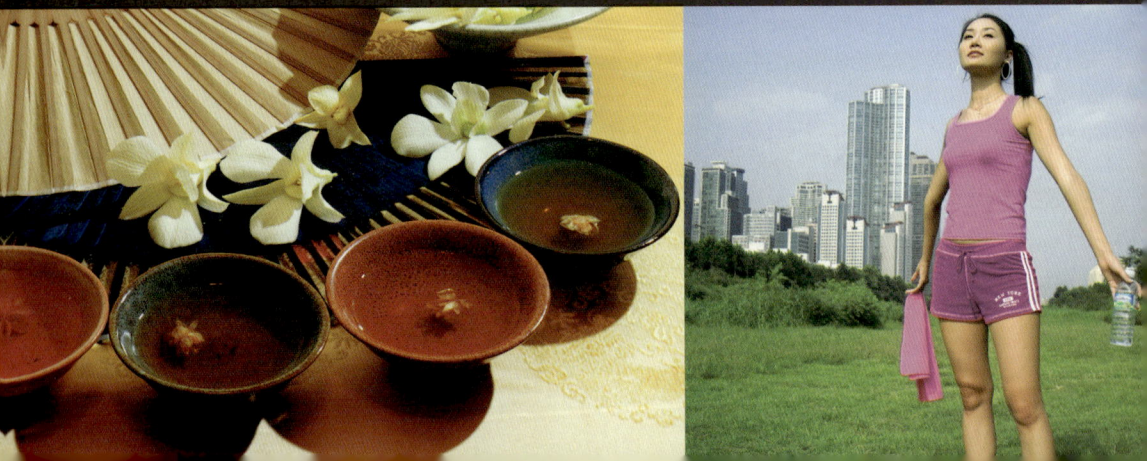

– Alice Walker

In order to invite someone into the magical realm of our soul and to share it with that special someone, the soul has to be made free and receptive, open to a cosmic union with another soul. The colour that works best when a person wishes to grow into the realm of a higher consciousness is not just one, but many including all shades of violet and indigo.

Violet, the colour possessing the shortest wavelength in the invisible electromagnetic spectrum stands for truth, deep introspection, friendship and communication with the higher energies. Historically, the colour purple has long been associated with royalty, perhaps because to produce the colour in ancient times was a time consuming and expensive task and only the elite could afford the use of the colour.

However, in modern times, not only is violet easily accessible but is found in almost everyone's wardrobe in some form or the other. This colour can be worn by a person to enable the mind to think freely. It also gives the wearer an enhanced sense of perception as well as a mystic understanding of one's inner spirituality. It is best to combine blue and violet to overcome stress and reduce tension because of their intrinsic tranquil qualities. It is also an ideal combination for those who wish to connect with the higher consciousness and aspire for spiritual awakening.

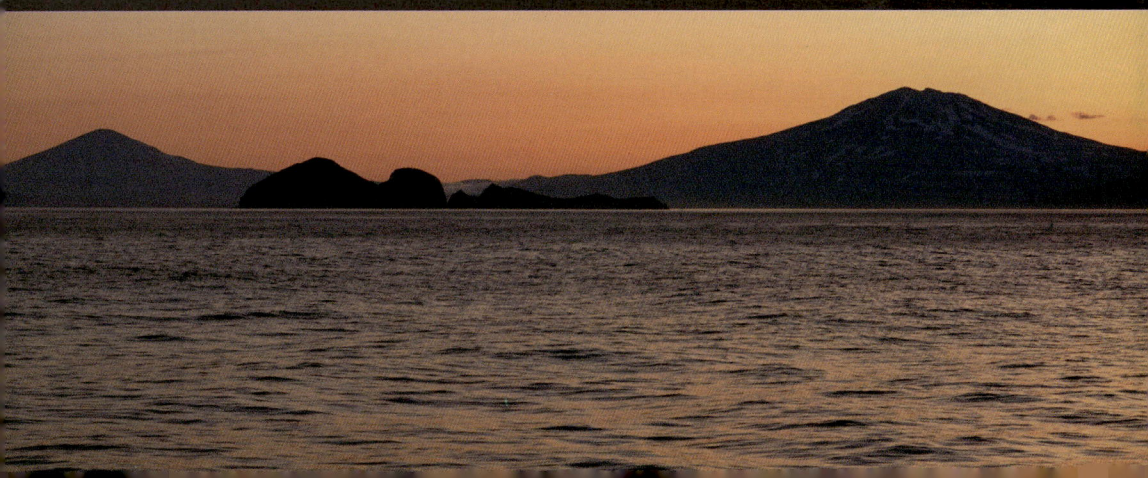

For a person who desires the magical feel of the colour purple as well as the warmth of emotions, it is best to combine violet and orange. Violet enables one to think and understand oneself and the world better, orange gets one talking which is ideal for most couples. As a person begins to discover his/her inner self, he/she will share the same experience with the partner due to the effect of orange.

Those who find violet a tad too dramatic a colour can tone it down by combining it with grey hues. This is considered by many, to be a very fashionable but under-used colour combination. Violet provides the wearer with a sense of peace where the mysticism becomes more transparent to the person and grey frees a person from emotional ties which inhibit a person from realizing their true inner feelings.

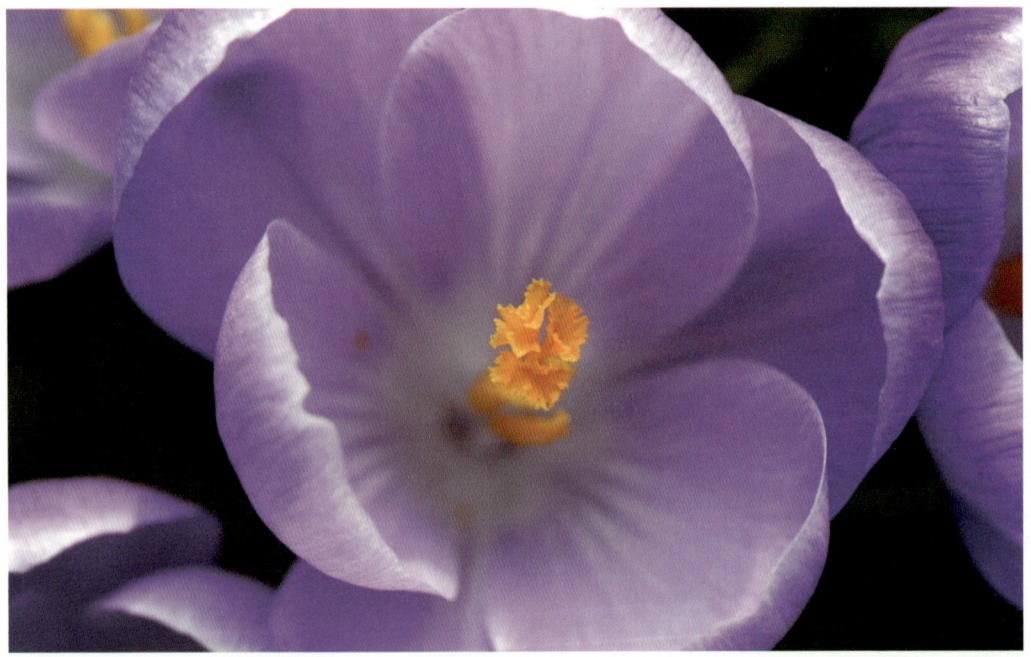

Violet calms the mind and rejuvenates the body and as such should be used in the interiors of the house in places where one wants solitude and serenity. It arouses a feeling of admiration within a person and he/she starts to appreciate others more.

Couples who want to be in perfect synchrony with each other's life must use violet or shades of it in their interiors in small but significant ways. For instance, purple upholstery greatly augments a room that has brown or wood tones in it. While brown, is a comforting colour that eases the nerves, purple creates an aura of magic and mysticism in the environment that sets the mood for a couple to undertake the journey of self realization by praying or meditating together.

Purple, combined with crimson and black is a classic colour scheme that works best in houses that convey class and elegance. While

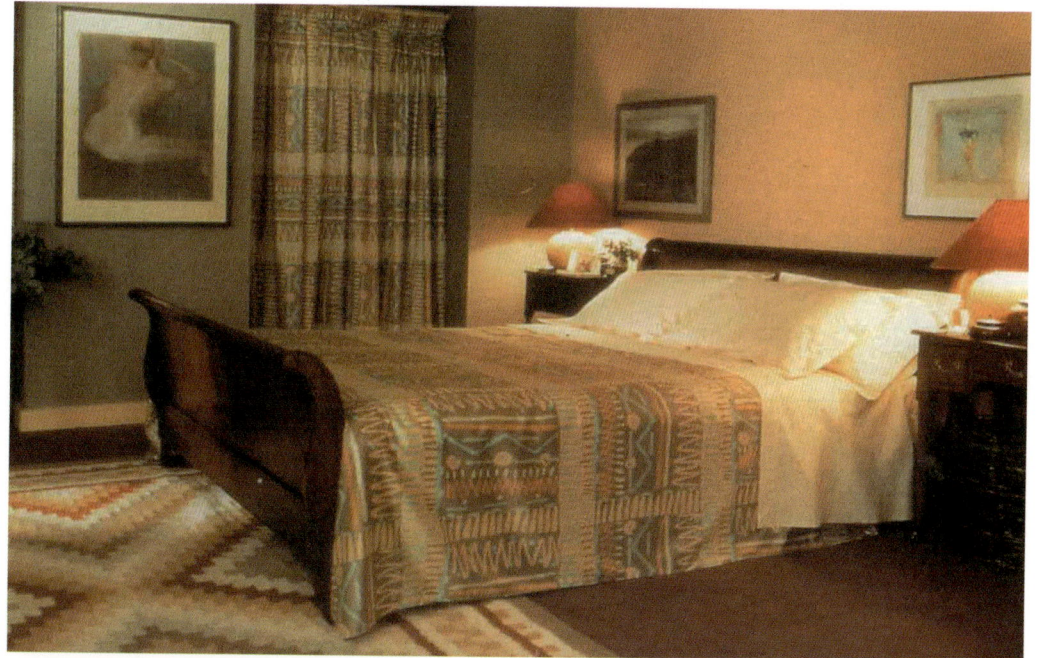

tones of violet create the vibrations most conducive to stimulating the spiritual nature of the people, black creates an atmosphere of perfect clarity and crimson stirs the passions. Due to the culmination of these three colours the couple indulges passionately in discovering each other by making the other a medium.

Another absolutely bizarre colour combination would be that of violet and gold. All shades of violet from mauve to purple blend harmoniously with the richness of colour. This is a dynamic combination since gold as a colour is seen to be magical in its own peculiar way. It expedites the effects of other

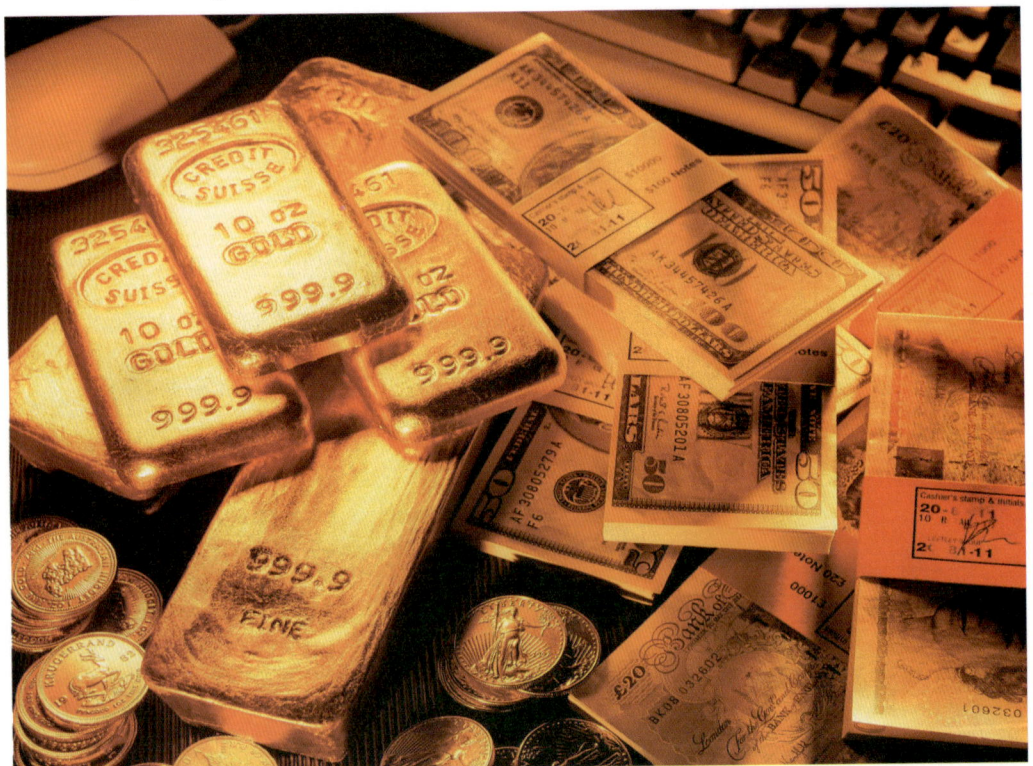

Towards a Healthy and Beautiful Relationship

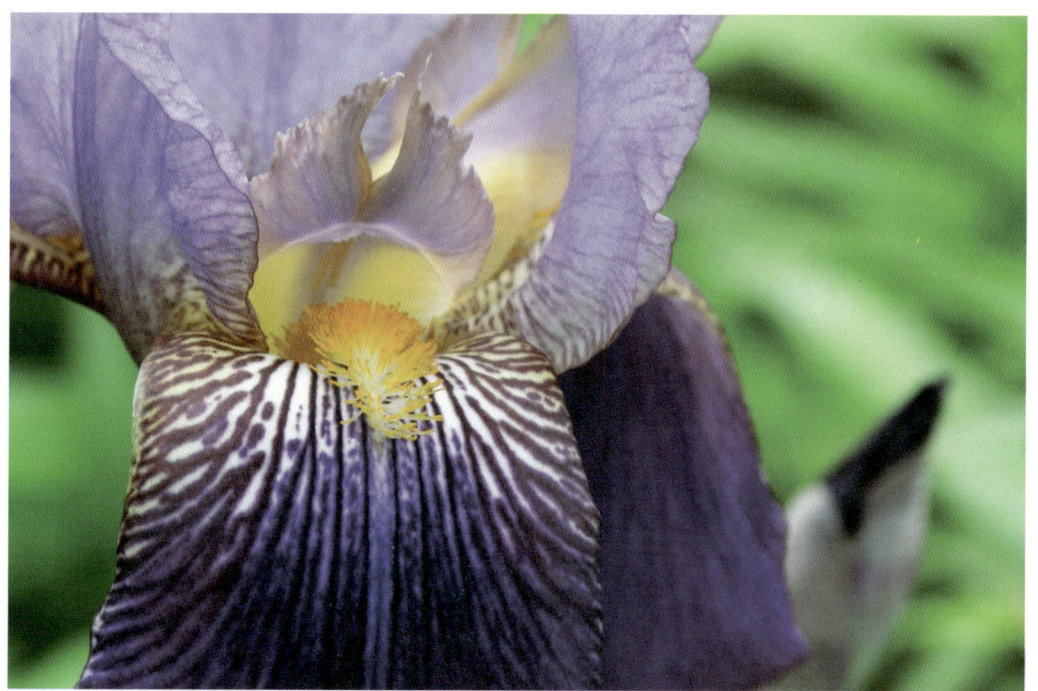

colours more than any other colour. Gold is also a warm colour that creates a sense of synchronization between two people's thoughts and ideas while violet plays its part in sharpening a person's intuition and insight. While the more dazzling tones of gold are attention grabbing, the soft, matte finish conveys sophistication and panache.

Another uncomplicated yet efficient way of incorporating the therapeutic qualities of violet in one's life is by taking a diamond shaped cardboard and painting it with a solid shade of purple or by sticking violet paper on it. This piece of cardboard can, then, be hung on a wall in the room or kept beside the bed and meditated upon for at least five minutes a day. This exercise helps in initiating the flow of the colour violet in the body and is just as effective in its therapeutic cure as painting the walls of a room or wearing violet coloured clothes.

Another simple way of assimilating the properties of purple in the body is by partaking purple foods like grapes, plums or eggplant and for those who love experimenting with food, here is a recipe worth trying:

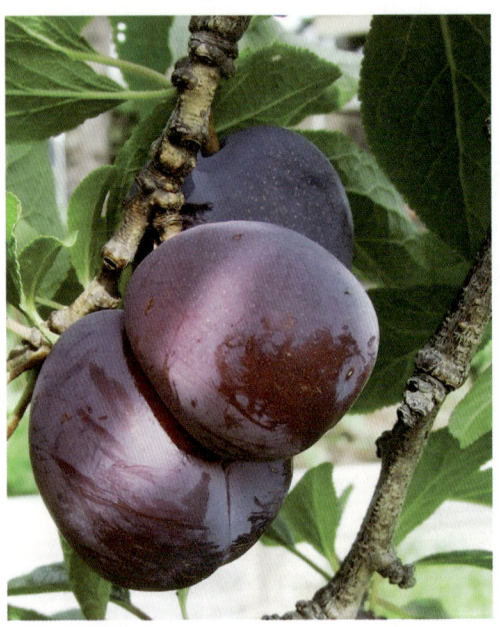

GOLDEN FRIED EGGPLANT SPREAD:

Ingredients:

- 1 large eggplant
- 2 tsp Chili Flakes
- 1 tbsp Coriander
- 1 tsp rosemary(optional)
- 1 tbsp whole wheat flour
- 1 egg
- Sea Salt to taste

Method:

Slice the eggplant thinly and pat dry. Brush the eggplant slices with the well- beaten egg and then dip the slices into a thick batter of flour and the spices. Fry the slices till golden brown and serve immediately.

Sometimes, one desperately wants to establish a spiritual connection with the partner for which the magic of candle therapy does wonders. The best candles to use are purple or any of its tints. A pillar candle or a candle encased in a jar can be used. To make this ritual effective, the couple should preferably light the candle when they are together with soft, soothing music, like the sounds of nature or the chime of bells, playing in the background.

Towards a Healthy and Beautiful Relationship

The candles should be lit in a dark place. The couple should dim all other lights so that the flame of the violet candle attracts all the focus. Then the couple should meditate upon the candle with the pure wish to know each other's soul. The rest works like magic and as, the days pass by, the mysticism of lighting the candle together will slowly come to light and the couple will find themselves melting and taking the shape

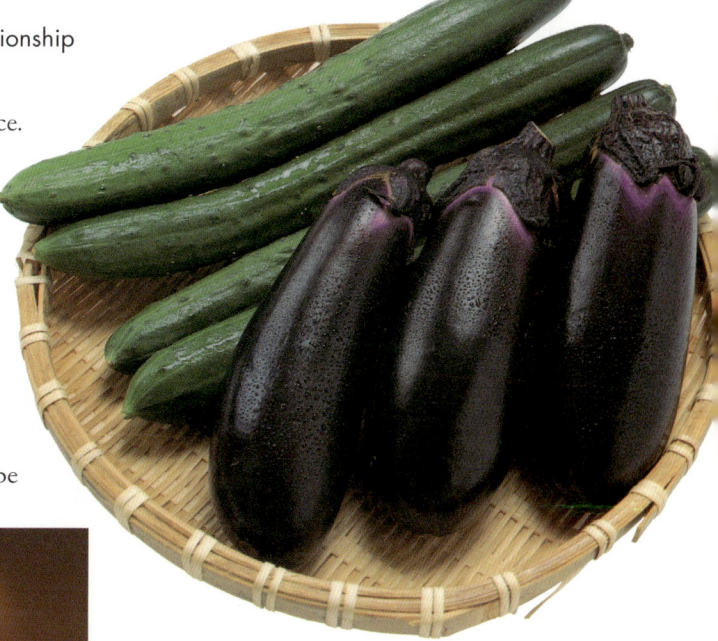

of the partner's personality.

Another simple technique of incorporating violet in one's life is by spiffing up all the interiors with violet flowers. Flowers, not only touch the heart and soul with their visual exquisiteness but also trigger the olfactory senses of the body, harmonizing all the senses and enveloping them with nature's own fragrances and untarnished beauty. The African lily is one such flower which stands majestic in its delicate splendour, almost demanding admiration. Its beauty not only enhances the surroundings but this flower can

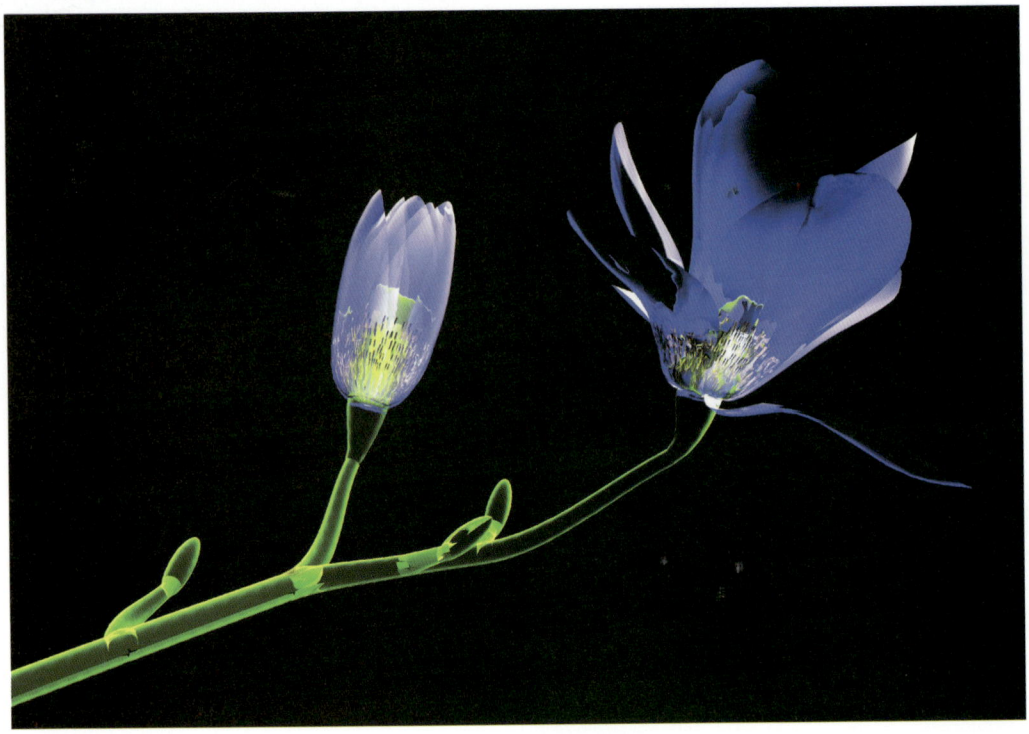

also be gazed upon to derive the qualities of this colour. Flowering onions and Canterbury bells are other examples of purple flowers.

An additional way of bringing in the delightful curative qualities of purple is by wearing shades of this colour. The purple-lensed glasses will help the body to absorb the colour through the eyes. Moreover, it doubles up as a fashion statement as well.

Violet can also be incorporated in one's daily life by breathing in this colour through a simple visualization exercise. This technique can be accomplished at any time when one is stress-free and peaceful, at dawn or when one

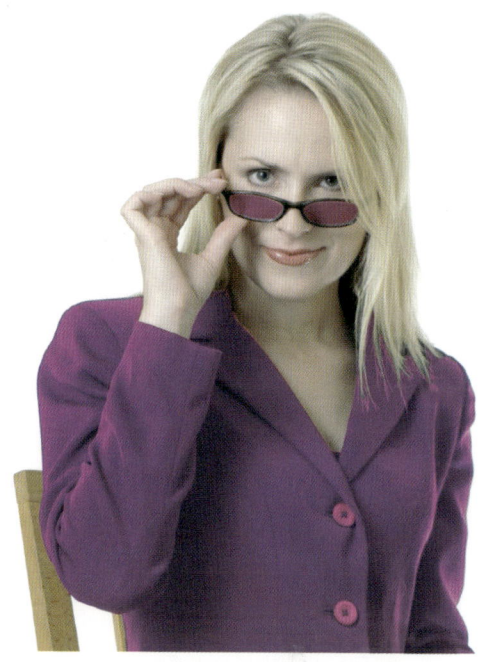

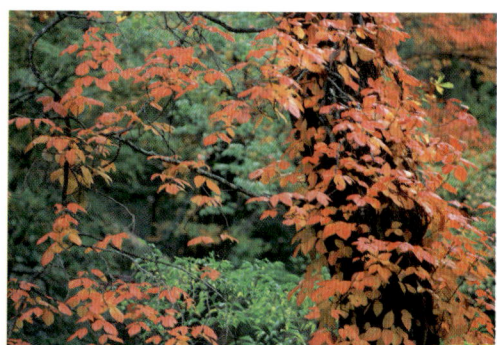

is ready to sleep. Sit or lie down in a relaxed position. Ensure that the body is warm and then begin to breathe in a natural and regular pattern.

Create in your mind an image of a beautiful garden full of your favourite flowers in bloom, exuding fragrances that you love. Visualize yourself walking through the garden bare foot. Feel the rays of the balmy sun upon yourself and as you walk in this blissful state, visualize that you have come across a beautiful church in the garden. Its walls are made of stained glass with appealing motifs and designs. Imagine yourself sitting in the church, appreciating its beauty. The sun rays filter in through the stained glass due to which all the purple motifs become bright.

Meditate upon this purple light. Imagine that the purple colour is seeping into every pore of your body as you sit inside the church. Continue this exercise as long as you feel

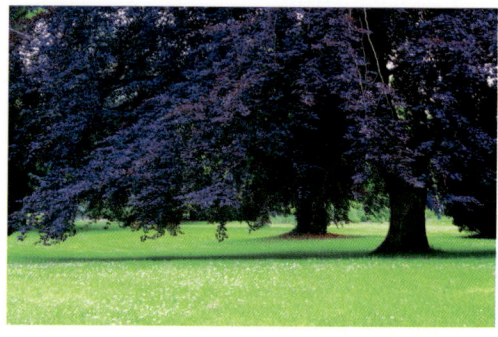

comfortable and then visualize yourself walking back from the church through the garden to your room where you have been meditating. Once you feel you are completely at ease with yourself, open your eyes slowly and remain still for a few minutes, taking in the surroundings of the room.

This particular visualization technique greatly assists people in balancing their inner selves with their social nature. The best results are assured when the couple does this technique together. It creates a sense of oneness not only during the exercise but even afterwards when they compare and assess their experiences.

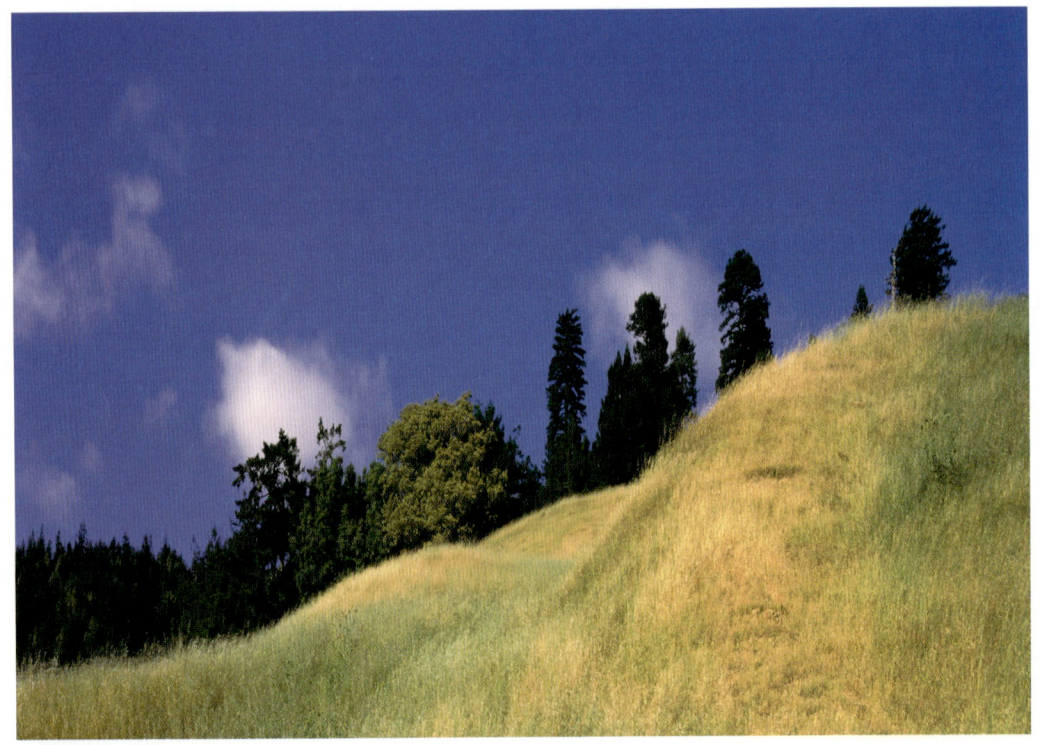

Towards a Healthy and Beautiful Relationship

A spiritual connection between two people can be established when they jointly involve themselves in activities, they are immersed in a unique feeling of oneness within themselves and with the divine energy of the cosmos surrounding them which can never be shattered.

Step 4: More than sex

Physical intimacy is one very important component of a relationship. As a couple begins to draw towards each other, a level of sexual closeness is achieved where the partners start exploring each other's, mind, body and soul and with it comes some of the best moments of a relationship.

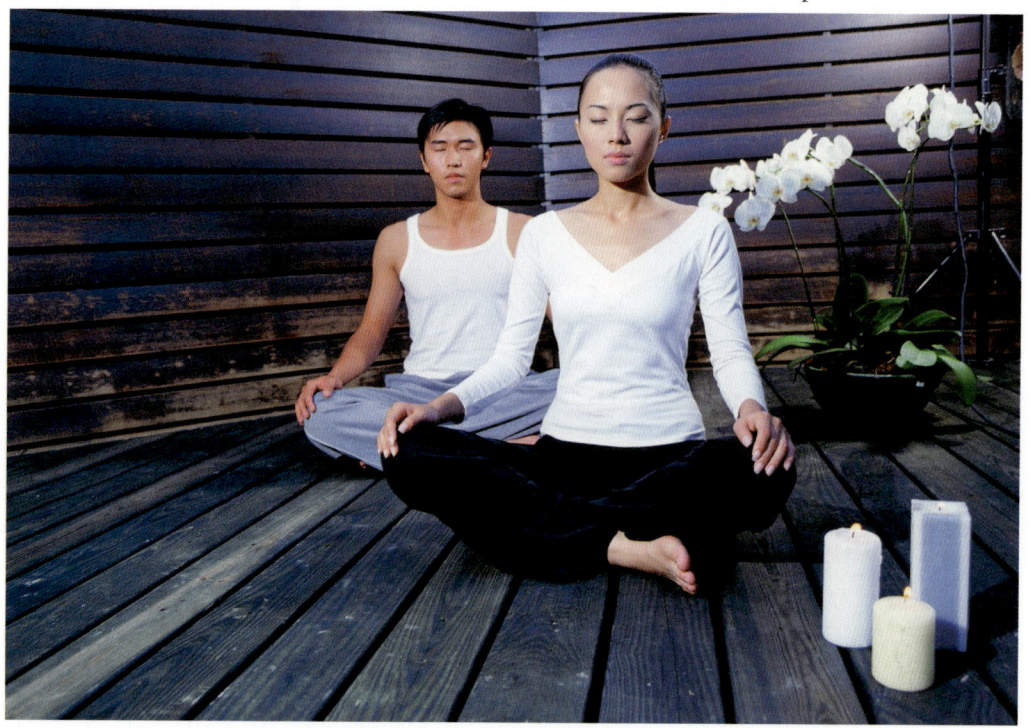

Physical proximity is not just about sex. It becomes a sacred act of discovering each other which is skin to a journey to the other person's soul through the realm of physical love. Many couples feel that there is a lot to be desired in the way of physical expression. Many are content with their love making but in both situations there is always scope of further enrichment and knowing the partner more intimately. This can be enhanced by the simple use of colours.

"I love red so much; I almost want to paint everything red". - Alexander Calder

When it comes to romance and intimacy, there is only one colour that comes to mind and rightly so: Red, the colour of love. This colour, supposedly the first to be perceived by man, is the colour of blood, of fire and everything else that denotes passion, heat and other intrinsically intense objects.

This is very effective in situations where passion needs to be aroused and the senses, stimulated. The first area where a couple can introduce this colour for better lovemaking is in the clothing section. When a couple feels in the mood for love or when even one partner's

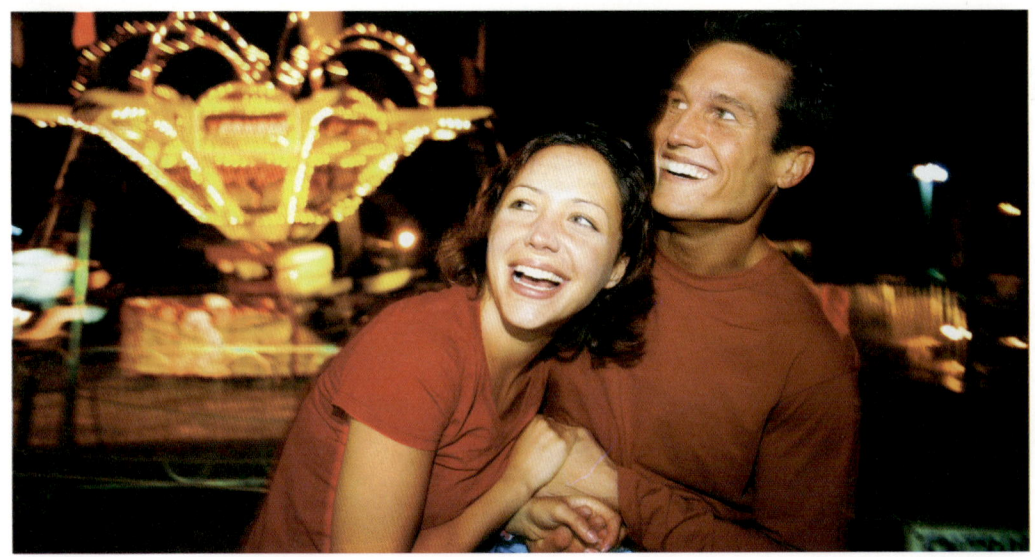

Towards a Healthy and Beautiful Relationship

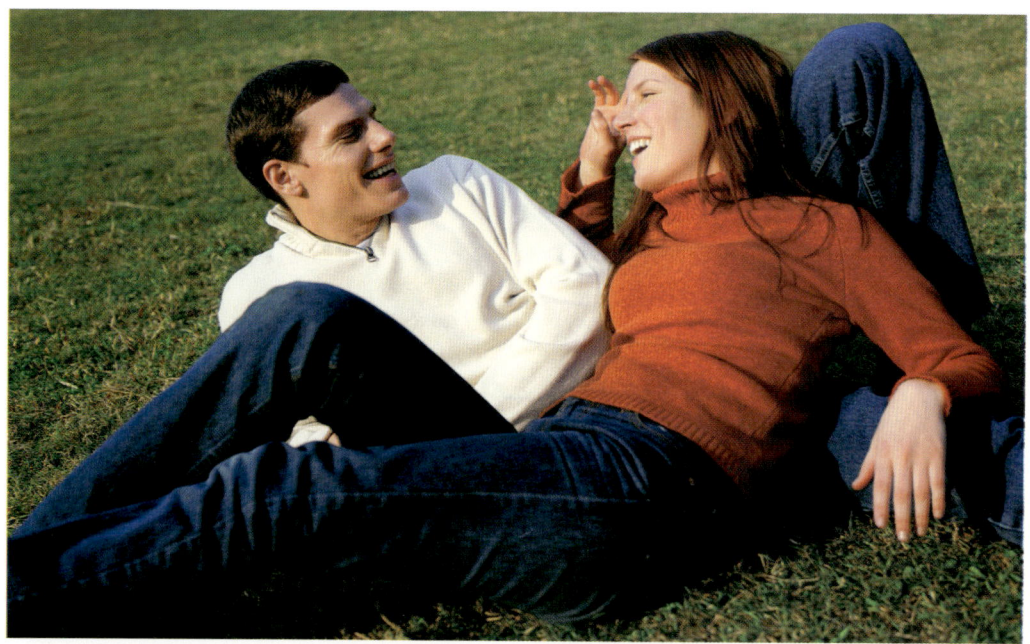

senses are ignited, the best thing to do is to wear red clothing. It not only energizes the partner who catches sight of the clothing but even the wearer feels motivated. The shades of red are many and a person should instinctively pick out what he/she is drawn to and it could be as racy as a tomato red to a more intense burgundy or crimson. Most couples are conservative about innerwear and not many are experimental with the colours. However, every couple should indulge in exciting innerwear in teasing shades of red to attract their partners and to have them completely mesmerized by the charms of love. There is a far greater choice of lingerie, in a plethora of styles, shades and textures for women, which will ensure a soul-stirring, unending journey of love making.

Red is known to make people lose track of time. That is just what a couple needs to enjoy; a long spell of making love. This colour can be made an intrinsic part of a couple's life by adding a dash of it to the interiors. A word of caution, red increases the respiration rate and the blood pressure of the body. Therefore, it is advisable to use red as a signature tone of the bedroom, albeit sparingly. Red should be used more as an accent colour and not as the base in the interiors.

Red works very well in rooms that are done up in a dark woody brown. It is a perfect complement to the look and adds a touch of panache to it. The darker tones of red like wine, crimson and burgundy add a touch of mystery when used with colours like lavender, purple or black. Red accents take on an earthy look when they are combined with brown shades like terracotta. When hues of red are combined with green and yellow, the room emanates a pulsating, vibrant feel.

Red can be added to the interiors in many ways. One can paint the walls with a combination of a central colour and red mixed to create a textured wall. While a high contrast combination will lend more energy to the room, a more subtle amalgamation will cause

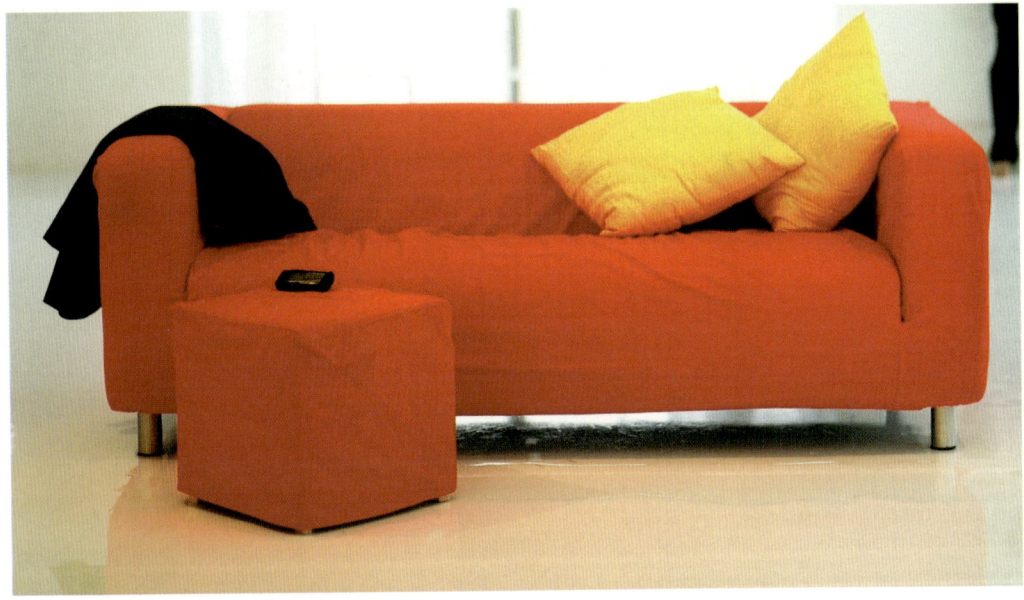

Towards a Healthy and Beautiful Relationship

the room to feel warm.

Another way to add red to the interiors is by painting the trims of the room in shades of red. Perhaps, just one wall, the door and window frames in red will do the trick. Red could be brought into the room by using red furniture which will stimulate and enrich the love making experience. It is advisable that the furniture should be comfortable since snug seating ensures cosiness.

Predominantly red paintings can be hung on the walls for the same effect. Some fine red paintings are Vincent Van Gough's 'The Red Vine', Piet Mondrian's ' Composition II- 1929',

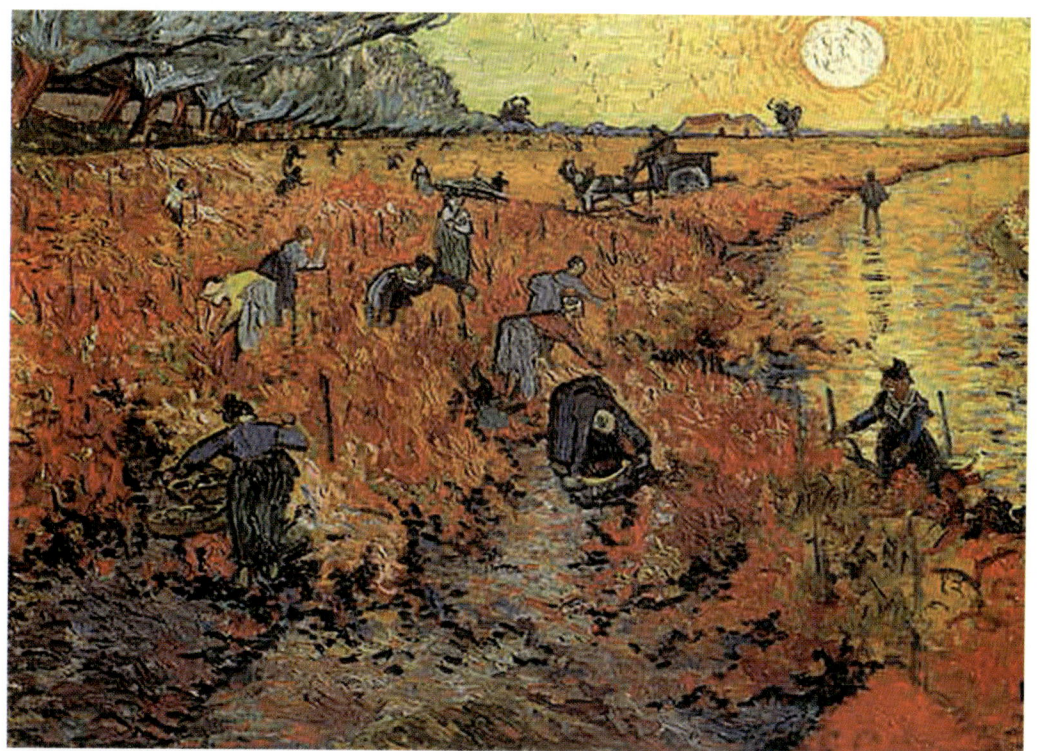

Kasimir Malevich's ' Head of a Woman' and Georgia O ' Keeffe's ' Red Gladiola in a White Vase'. For many the red walls or furniture might seem too loud. Such people can add red vases or ornaments in the room. According to Feng – Shui, anything that adorns the room of a couple must be in pairs, for instances, candle stands, two similar picture frames or a pair of mandarin ducks or fish which enhances the positivism of the room. If any of these are in hues of red, the couple avails of the dual benefits of colour therapy and Fen –Shui.

Upholstery or carpets are an equally effective way of bringing in red to rooms. Red curtains add both movement and energy to the room. Red bed sheets are a good idea too. Red candles particularly the pillar variety, being enormous, add red to the interiors and can be placed strategically around the bedroom not only to lend the desired aura of red to the room but also to create the mood for perfect love making, when lit.

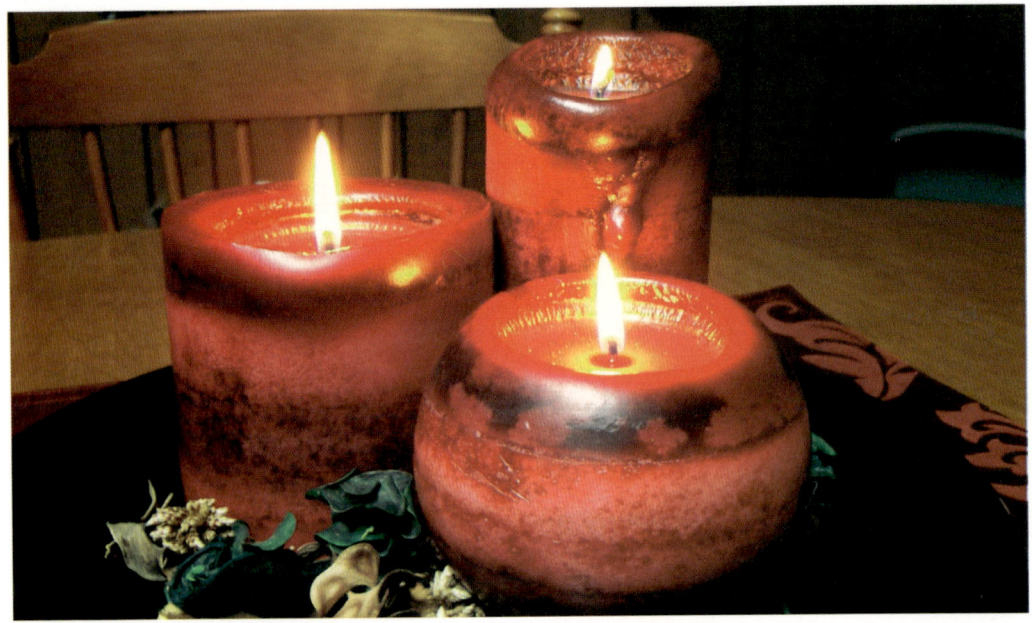

Certain scents corresponding to the colour red, can be used to imbibe the qualities of this intense colour without having to visually absorb it in the body.

One of the most popular red scents is rose. The petals of this flower are used to extract the rich aromatic oil and its aroma is believed to quell all disagreements and bring upon a feeling of love and warmth. This is a rich and intense fragrance found commonly in essential oils, bathing gels, shampoos, perfumes and soaps as well. It is known to have an aphrodisiacal effect on those who use it.

Another exotic 'red' scent is that of cinnamon. Most commonly used in India, Japan and Burma, this particular fragrance, much like the rose, is considered to possess aphrodisiacal qualities and when used as incense or in the form of scented candles, the aroma creates an inviting and erotic mood. Cinnamon is used in Chinese medicine to treat colds and impotence and is known to fuel fantasies, just the right element to add to a budding romance.

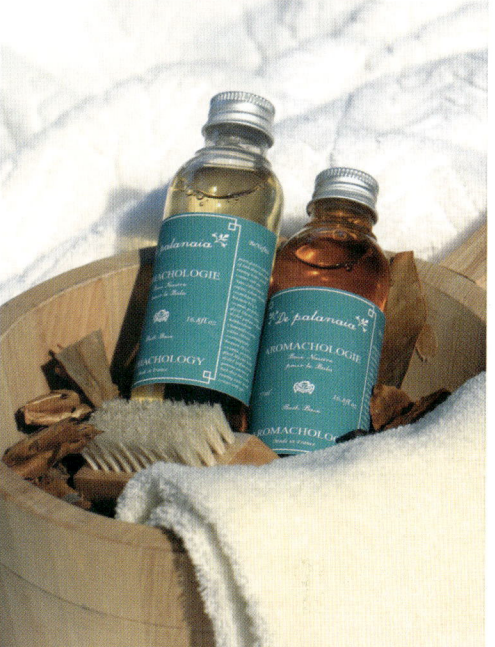

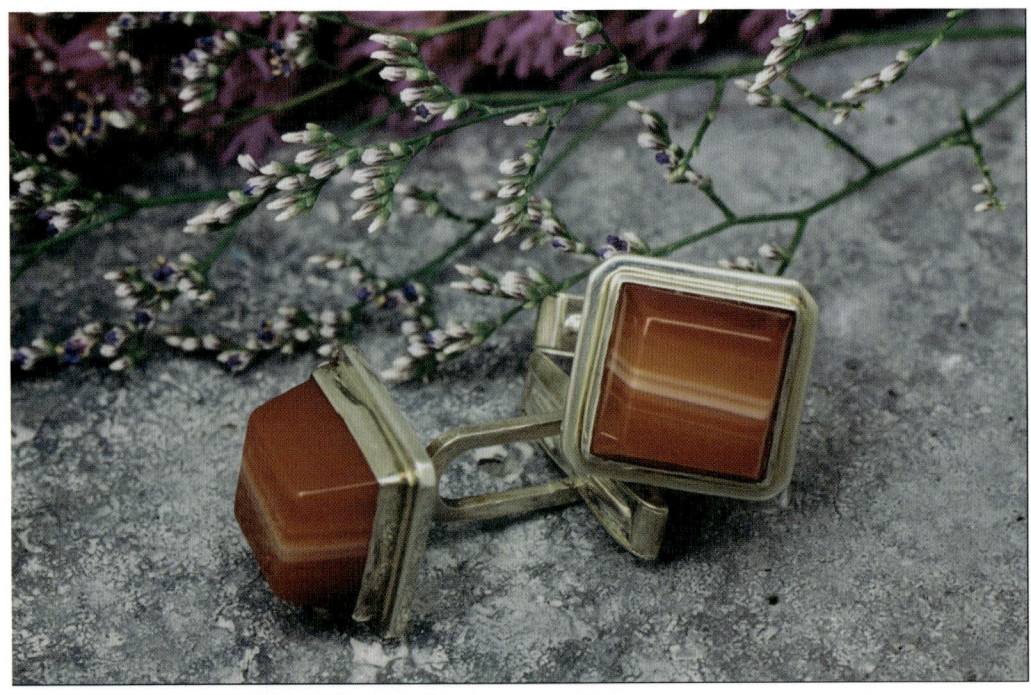

The dynamic characteristic of red is also found in the scent of pine. According to German folklore, the scent of pine acts as a shield against negative energies. Not only is this scent energizing, but is also useful when people wish to bury the problems from their past and make a fresh beginning. This scents works wonders for couples who are trying to bring the romance back to their lives and it gives a new lease of life to their lovemaking as well.

For those who like everything spicy, from their lives to their lovemaking, the fragrance of ginger, which corresponds to the colour red, is an interesting option. According to Greek folklore, it was used in ancient Greece to reduce the effects of poison. Its fragrance is known to ease mood swings and open up blocked channels of energy within a person, which in turn enhances communication between a couple. This is a hot and pleasing aroma, considered one of the seven important incense substances as prescribes by Zen Buddhism.

All the above fragrances are available in the form of incense as well as essential oils and they can be diluted in water and then heated in an oil burner to permeate all over. Another method of using the scent is to have one partner massage the other's body with the oils, in these fragrances. Rose and pine are even used as main ingredients of shower gels and these gels can be used by a couple to enjoy a heady shower together that will enhance their sensual instincts and get them in the mood for some erotic lovemaking.

The romantically evocative qualities of the colour red can be derived from various natural gemstones that can be worn in the form of rings, bracelets and neckpieces. Each gemstone has its own unique properties that can greatly enhance the love and romance quotient in one's life.

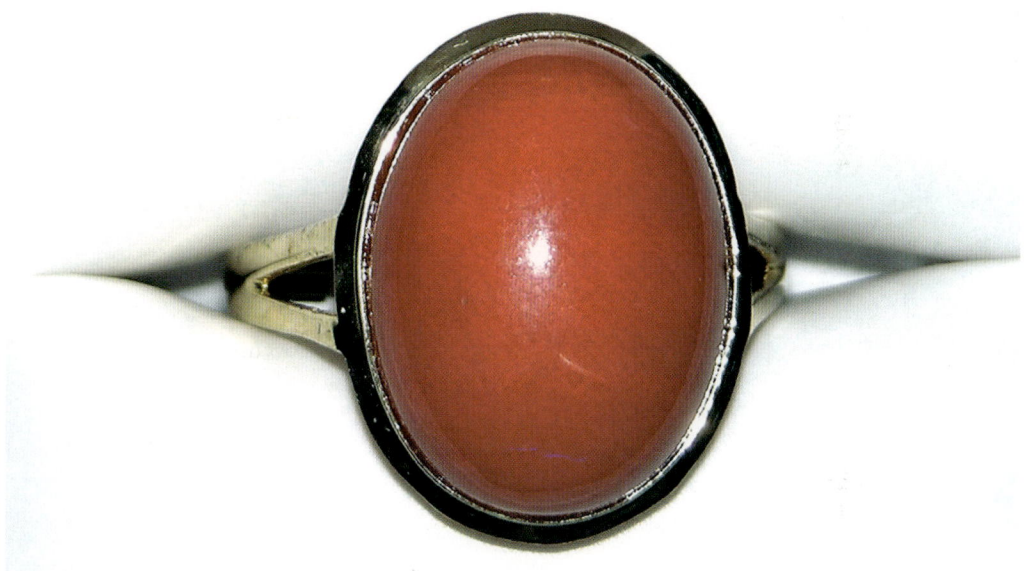

Red Jasper is one such stone which not only adds vitality to the wearer's body but also fortifies his/her physical energy as well as the consciousness. In addition, it keeps the bloodstream clean and detoxified, making the circulatory system healthy and strong.

There is the red Garnet. Garnets are found in all colours except blue. It must necessarily be the red variety. However, if the gemstone is used for love and passion, it is known by all that wearing a red garnet promotes sincerity and devotion in the wearer and also augments the energy levels of those wear it, while dispelling negative vibrations from the body.

Another stone that is commonly found in nature in its yellow hue but every now and then nature proffers its red form as well, is Topaz. This stone when worn in its red shade, dispels grief and anguish, bestowing upon its wearer newfound fecundity and a positive

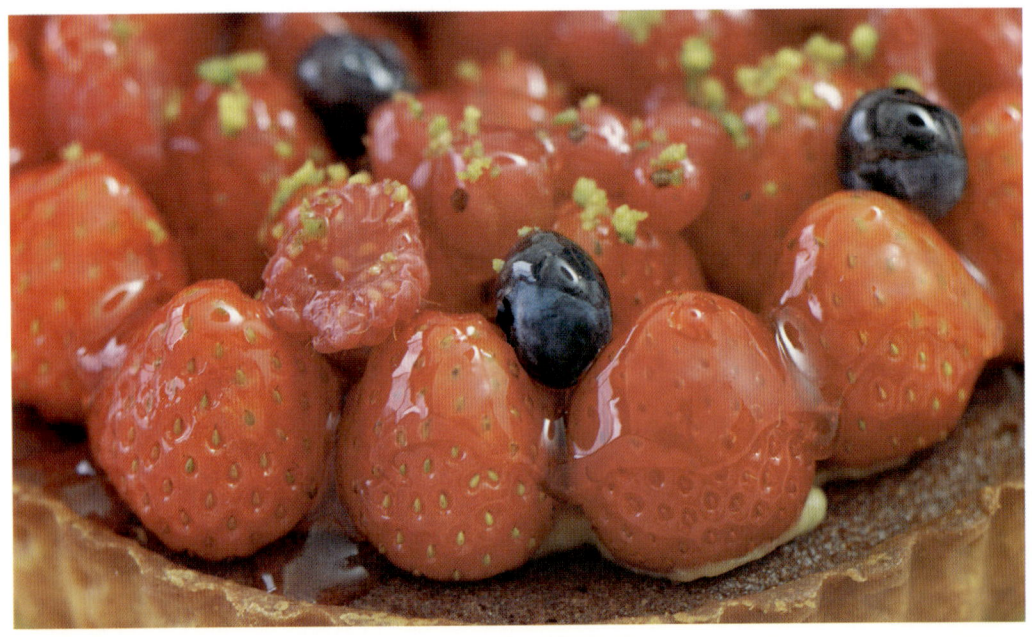

frame of mind. It energizes the mind and body of the wearer significantly. It is reputed to enhance the looks of those who wear it. Then there is Ruby which is considered one of the most precious gemstones on this planet. Derived from the Latin word 'Rubens', the word Ruby literally means red and one can imagine what a punch it packs. The red of this stone is fiery, passionate and fervent, stirring up the same feelings in the one who wears it. It fires the passion in a relationship adding to its strength and ardour, the best ingredients to a perfect romance! It is beneficial to incorporate red food items in one's daily meal. Red food as an option to add more fiery red to a relationship works tremendously well. Not only do red foods and vegetables promote vitality and synergy but also paves a way to one's heart. There are many red foods available that can not only lend their curative properties to a romancing couple, but can also be used as a part of foreplay, to add that special zing to lovemaking. The variety of such foods is endless; the top contenders on the list include strawberries, watermelon and cherry tomatoes. To spice things up a bit more, there's always the deliciously red Virgin Mary for the experimental one.

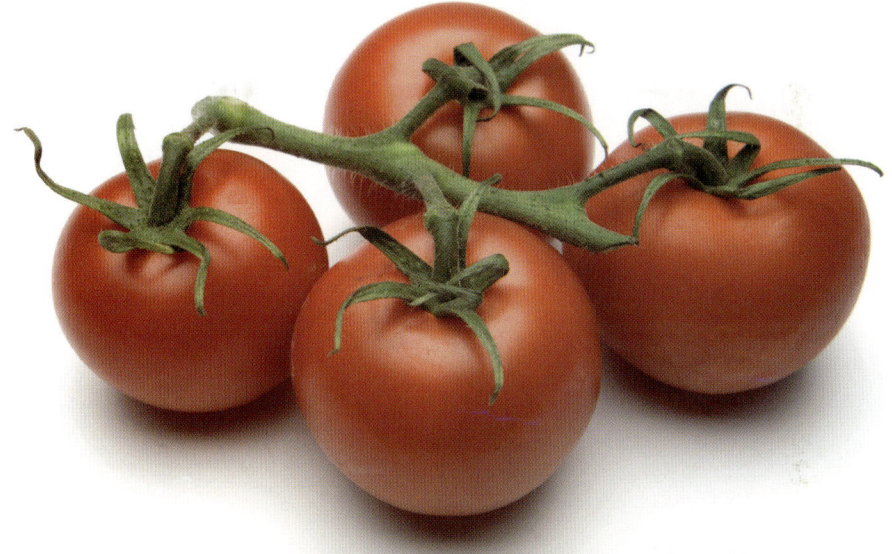

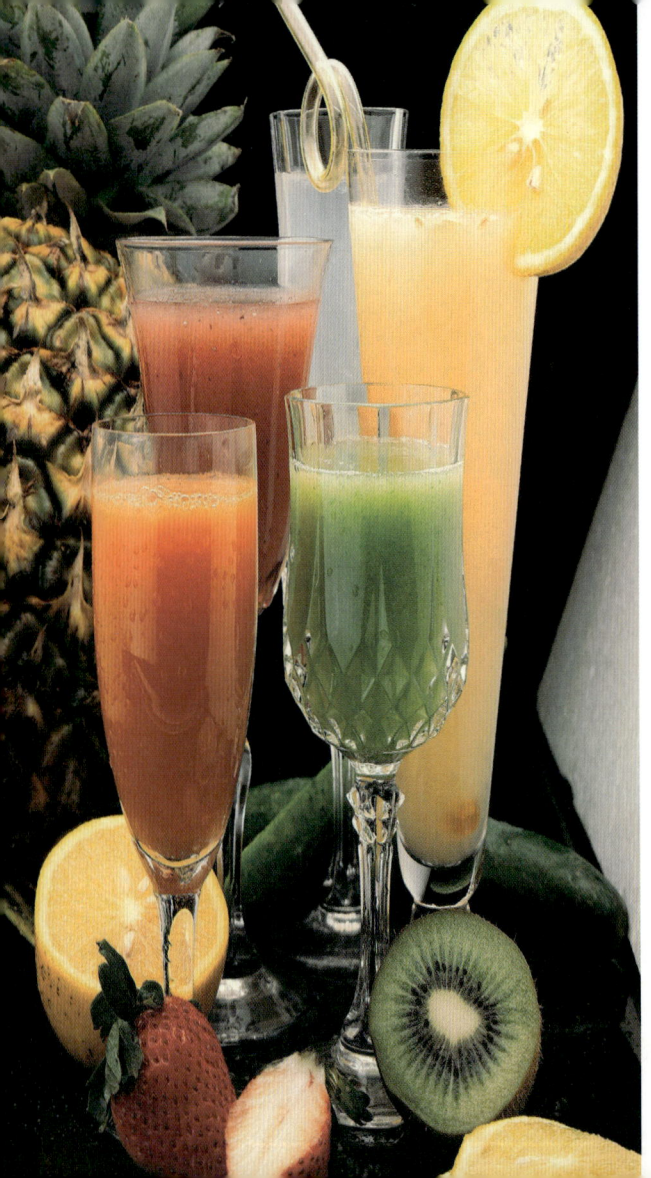

Colour Therapy for Love & Romance

Ingredients:
- 2 Cups Tomato Juice
- 4 drops Tabasco Sauce
- 5 drops Worcestershire Sauce
- 4-5 dashes lemon juice
- 1 pinch celery salt
- 1 pinch ground pepper

Method:

Pour the tomato juice over ice cubes in a tall glass, season and stir. Ready to serve in bed!

Music and making love traditionally go together. The right ambience and sensual music can render lovemaking an unforgettable experience. One can choose to further heighten passion.

Red music is what relates to the note of C in the middle octave of the musical spectrum. Such music stimulates the mind and body, lending to it a rhythm of vigour and passion, building up intensity within the body and creating a frenzied rhythm between two bodies.

Examples of red music are Franz Schubert's 'Moments Musical', No# 1 in C major, Mozart's 'Piano Sonata' No.10 in C and Deepak Chopra's 'Desire' (Sex Lounge – Part1).

Chapter 7
BREAKING UP

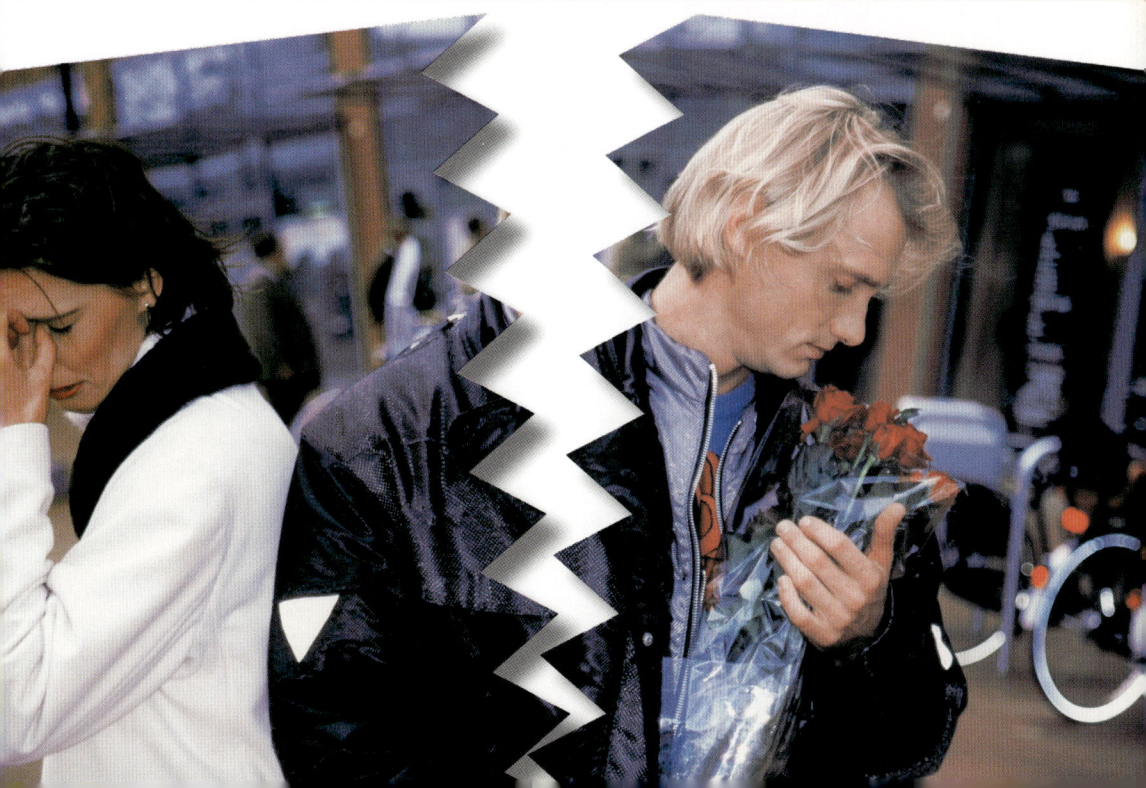

Love is a beautiful experience but it also tends to hurt just as much when it's over. It leaves one totally shattered and clueless about how to begin life afresh. The first step to healing is to realize that all is not lost. One must take stock of the situation and decide upon the direction to be taken. Slowly but steadily, things will fall into place and life will move on- initially with a lot of pain, but for the better.

'Green is the fresh emblem of well – founded hopes. In blue, the spirit can wander, but in green, it can rest' – Mary Webb

The first step towards dealing with a break up is to find the energies of our physical and emotional being and internalize them, in order to commence harmonizing them and giving ourselves renewed vigour and the courage to carry on, with motivation and the belief that life holds greater opportunities for us. Green can be included in one's life through the interiors of the room in which one spends maximum time. Visual contact with this colour ensures that the body assimilates its healing powers effectively. Another good thing about adding this colour to the interiors is that it brings the outdoors inside the house which will naturally have a therapeutic effect on whoever sits in the room for long periods of time.

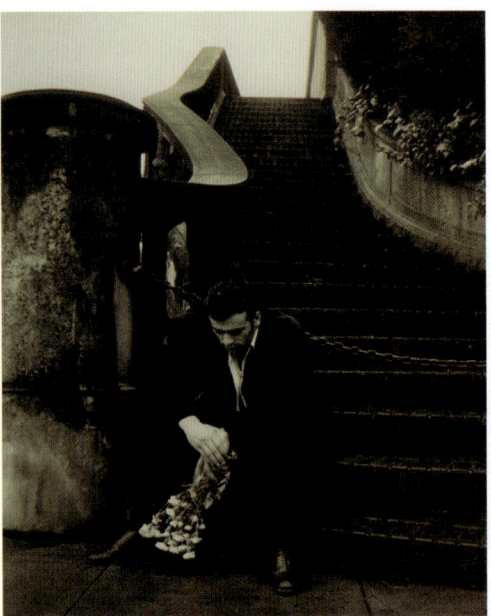

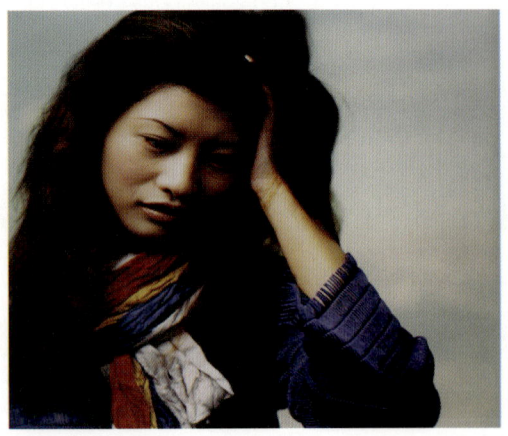

There are many shades and hues of green to choose from. Depending on the tone of green, it can be combined with various other colours for a dual effect. On its own, the lighter shades of green like olive and sage are good options to lend a serene and pleasing feel to the room.

The darker shades of green can be combined with a rich burgundy, an intense but subtle gold and even the classic black to add opulence to a room at the same time reinforcing the stability factor. This is because all these colours combine to give a very secure and stable feel to both the room as well as

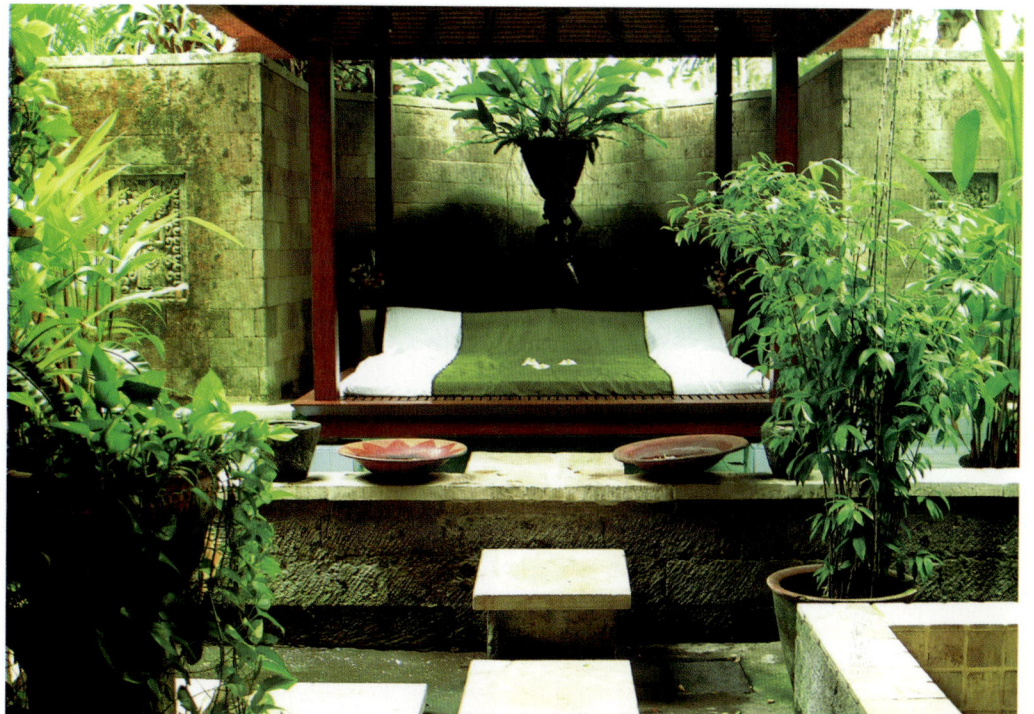

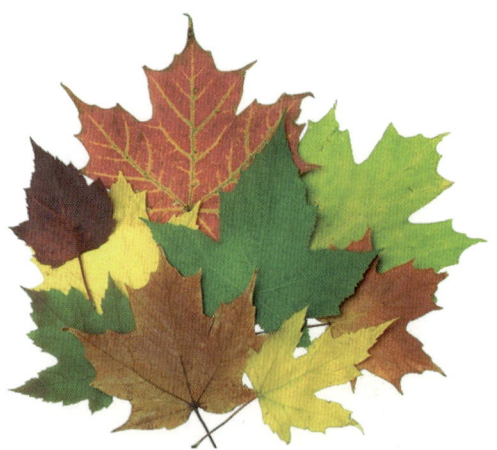

those who spend time there.

For those who like green in its pop avatar, can use chartreuse: a lively colour indeed but can get on to the nerves if not used sparingly as an accent. This particular shade of green can be combined with yellow to bring in that sunny feeling that adds to the comfort quotient of the room. Yellow enhances one's mental clarity while green rejuvenates a tired mind and body. Chartreuse can also be paired with magenta to add mega power to the room. With this combination, it is impossible to feel low.

Painting the walls of a room green is not the only way one can bring in its therapeutic qualities to a room: green accents across a room have the same effect. What really helps while doing up a room is to remember that there should be apparent unity of design and colour in the room. There should be places like the window sill, the photograph corner or even a fireplace, which must be emphasized and other areas which need to be underplayed.

Green bed covers along with green curtains can be used in the bedroom. The living room can be done up in a refreshing green upholstery with another colour thrown in to break the monotony. Beautiful rugs in various shades of green can be spread about to add movement and character to a room. Green lampshades, placed strategically help to create the desired mood in the room.

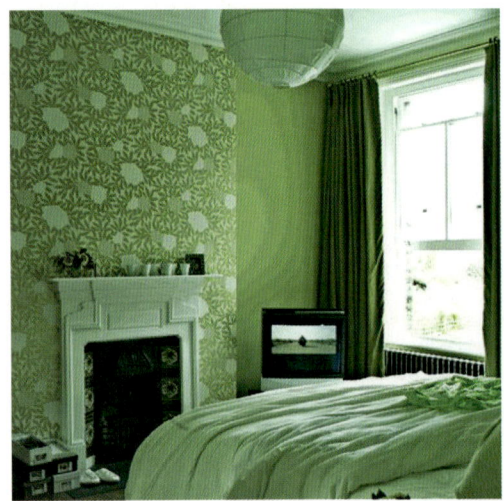

Breaking up

Another option is to use green pillar or glass encased candles all over the room for a magical effect .As enhancements, their visual beauty is astounding. When lit, they create an atmosphere of peace and harmony which, in turn, help a person to focus on his inner revitalization.

Those who wish to make minimal changes in their rooms and yet achieve the effects of green, can opt for paintings that are largely green and which must be hung where they are most visible .Examples of such paintings, reproductions or prints of which can easily be sourced are Pablo Picasso's 'Jacqueline with a cat', Claude Monet's 'White Water Lilies' and even photographs of nature in all its splendour

When talking about green, it's not only getting the outdoors inside. One can get the same advantage of green if one has a verandah or a garden around the house. This part of the house can be converted into nature's paradise by planting exotic plants and trees. This will not only make the environs rich but gardening and tending to plants is therapeutic also. It lends peace and quietude to the one who chooses to meditate in this manner. The garden can be developed as a theme, with a specific colour pattern, with herbs, birdbaths-the possibilities are limitless. Apart from

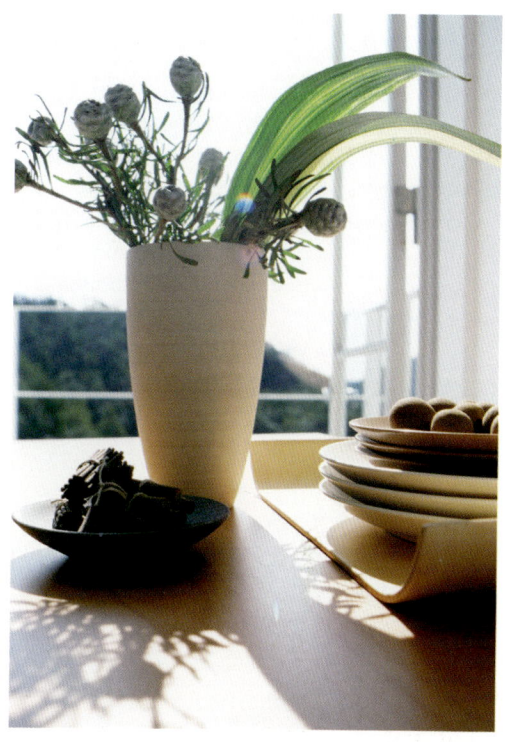

adding beauty to the home, it enables one to divert the mind from various problems.

A stylish way to absorb the colour green is to wear sunglasses with green tints. There is a wide range of green-tinted glasses available in the market. When light filters in through the green-tinted glasses, it has the same therapeutic effect on the mind and body as using green for the interiors.

One can assimilate the benefits of green by eating foods which are green in colour. The range of such foods is limitless. There is something green for every taste. Moreover, cooking by itself is therapeutic in nature. By the time the cooking is over, the person is less distressed and more in harmony with one's inner self.

MIXED GREENS:
Ingredients:

- 1 beetroot
- ½ cabbage
- ½ cup chopped spinach
- ½ cup chopped string beans
- Seasoning to taste

Method:

Place a heavy saucepan on the flame. Put 1 tablespoon olive oil and add the ginger and garlic paste. Sauté it for a few seconds. Add the chopped vegetables along with the seasoning. Toss and stir constantly over high flame for 3-5 minutes till the vegetables are slightly tender. Serve immediately.

There are many essential oils and fragrances corresponding with the colour green that can assist one by taking away the grief and agony caused by a breakup.

Cinnamon is one of the most effective green essential oil which is often used to cure arthritis and infections. This oil has a very calming effect on the mind and body but as an essential oil it cannot be recommended as massage oil. Instead, it can be heated in a diffuser to fill the environment with

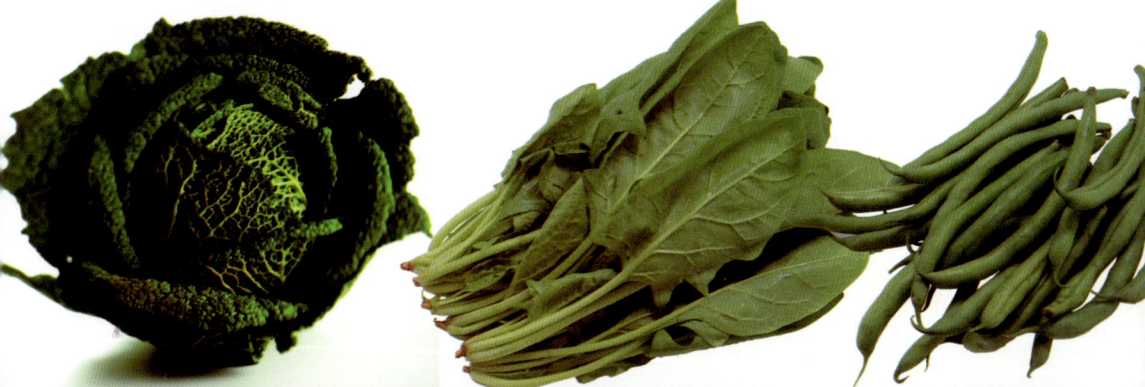

Breaking up

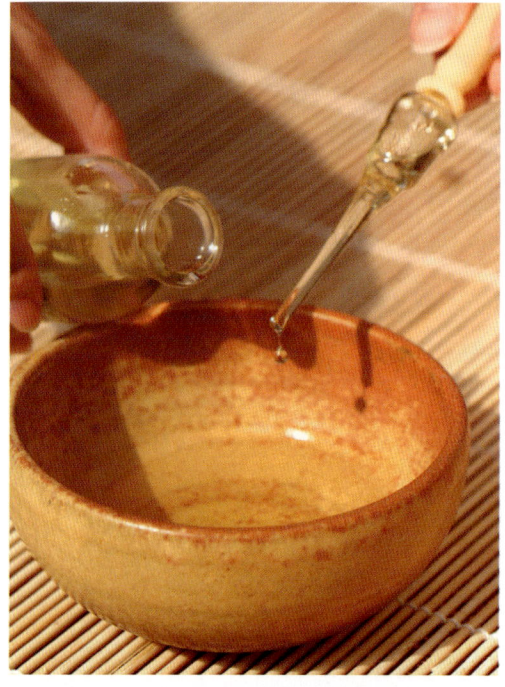

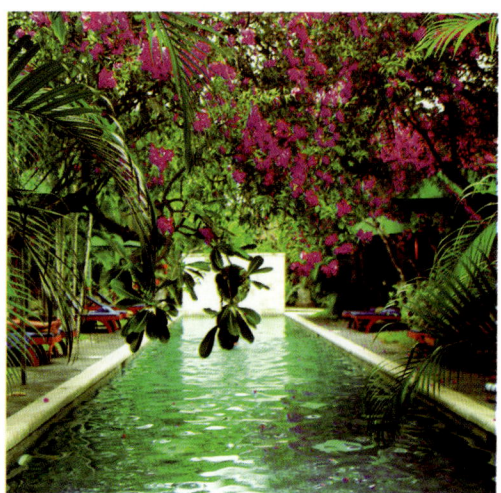

a compelling fragrance which promotes harmony and equilibrium in life.

Cinnamon is found in many kinds of incense and its use can be traced back to ancient Egypt and Greece where it was used as a healing aroma for years. Burning it as an incense will create a warm and inviting atmosphere that will trigger a sense of liberation within a person and slowly dispel all pent up distress, replacing it with serenity and quietude.

Neroli is another oil which is effective in helping a person deal with a break up. Made from the blossoms of the orange tree, it has a sweet and floral fragrance that engulfs the consciousness of a person. It relieves the mind and soul of despair and strain. It is often used in bridal bouquets to be able to soothe the bride's frazzled nerves.

If looking for incense that lends a green aura to the room, camphor is an excellent choice. Camphor is found as a primary ingredient in many forms of incense and it can also be burnt in its crystalline form. Camphor has been used in India since time immemorial.

Ayurveda incorporates its curative properties to treat anxiety and hysteria. The strong and all-engulfing aroma of camphor facilitates the opening up of the five senses lending a feeling of emancipation and giving one the courage to move ahead.

The dual combination of Marjoram and Lavender essential oils correspond with green and are exotic as well. Marjoram is widely used by aroma therapists around the world for its sedating qualities. It fills one with a sense of calm. Marjoram blends well with lavender, another extract that enjoys a primary status amongst essential oils. This oil is derived from exquisite purple flowers. It has a soothing effect on the mind, owing to its fresh and warm fragrance. Not only does it enhance a sense of harmony and balance, but is also known to be just as soothing for the skin.

Green gemstones assist greatly by calming one's nerves apart from looking stunning. The green gemstones that can be used for their

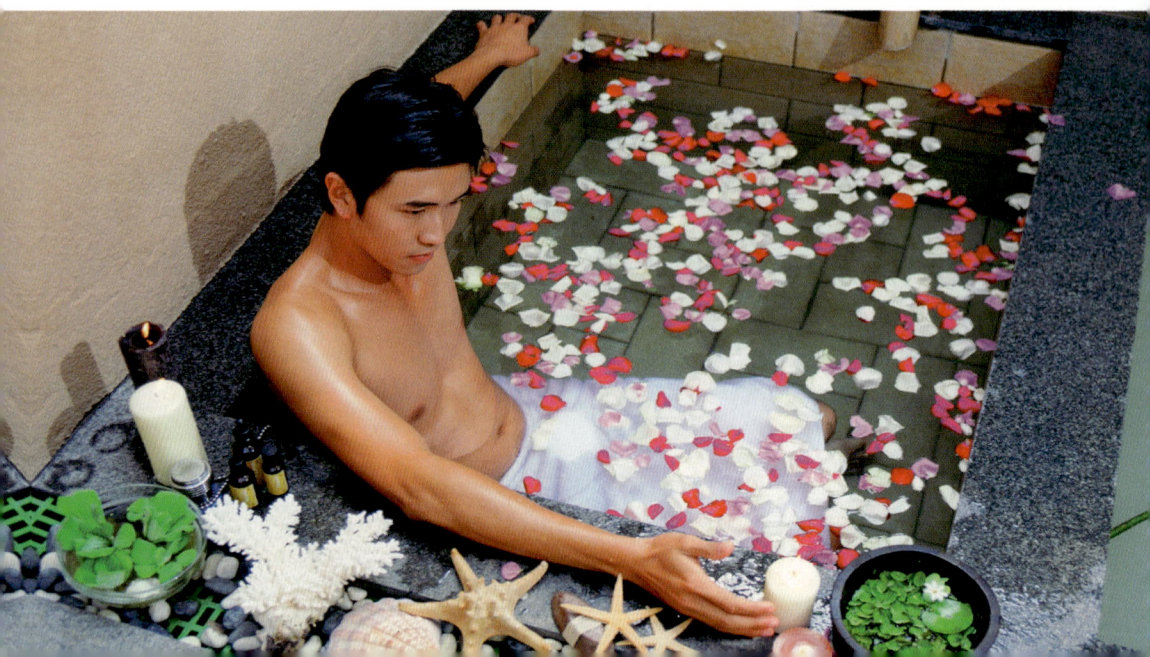

Breaking up

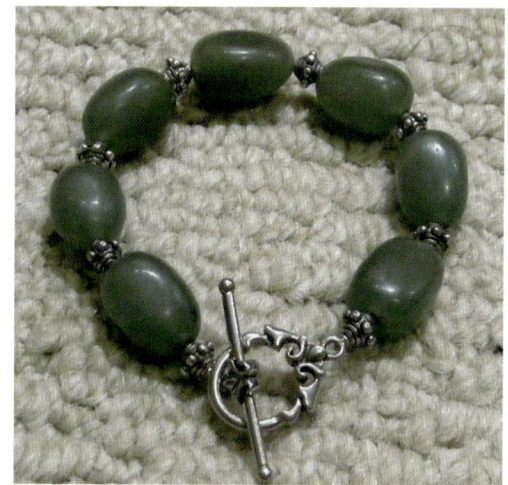

therapeutic properties are varied. One such example is Green Calcite. This stone not only enables one to break free from shackles of past hurt but also propels the transition from a negative state of mind to a more positive and fulfilling one.

Lime green is yet another green stone that assists greatly in dealing with the trauma of a break up. This stone induces calmness in the wearer and also cleanses the emotional plane, detoxifying the mind and leading to a positively energized frame of mind.

Aventurine is yet another green stone found in nature that brings tolerance, balance and prosperity to the wearer of the stone. This gemstone is particularly beneficial for the distressing times like a break up; since it is known to spiritually shield the heart from hurt and suffering. Its other effective facet is that it helps dissolve emotional blockages in the system, thereby giving the wearer a feeling of emotional liberation.

No one can deny the therapeutic qualities of music. There is ' Green Music' that relates to the key of ' F' in the musical spectrum and is known to balance the rhythms thereby calming the mind and body. This music is soothing and invigorating for positive thoughts to start flowing in the heart. Listening to it for as little as fifteen minutes can greatly help soothe an anxious or distressed mind.

Some fine examples of green music are 'Hari Om' by Ravi Shankar found in the album ' Chants of India', ' Accepting Tranquillity' by Talveen Singh, ' Claire de Lune' by Debussy and ' Fairy King' by Mike Rowland.

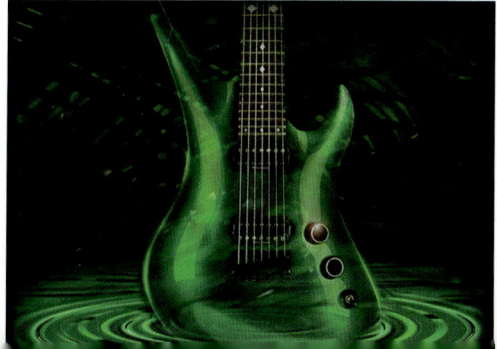